Complete SAQs
for Medical Finals

09

DATE DUE FOR RETURN

This book may be recalled before the above date.

Complete SAQs for Medical Finals

Philip Stather MBChB
University Hospitals of Leicester, UK

Helen Cheshire MBChB
University Hospitals of Leicester, UK

Joanna Manton MBChB BSc (Hons)
University Hospitals of Leicester, UK

Mahul Gorecha MBChB
University Hospitals of Leicester, UK

WITH SENIOR ADVISER
Tania Riera MB BChir MA MRCGP
General Practitioner

WILEY-BLACKWELL

A John Wiley & Sons, Ltd., Publication

This edition first published 2010, © 2010 by Philip Stather, Helen Cheshire, Joanna Manton, Mahul Gorecha and Tania Riera

Blackwell Publishing was acquired by John Wiley & Sons in February 2007. Blackwell's publishing program has been merged with Wiley's global Scientific, Technical and Medical business to form Wiley-Blackwell.

Registered office: John Wiley & Sons Ltd, The Atrium, Southern Gate, Chichester, West Sussex, PO19 8SQ, UK

Editorial offices: 9600 Garsington Road, Oxford, OX4 2DQ, UK
The Atrium, Southern Gate, Chichester, West Sussex, PO19 8SQ, UK
111 River Street, Hoboken, NJ 07030-5774, USA

For details of our global editorial offices, for customer services and for information about how to apply for permission to reuse the copyright material in this book please see our website at www.wiley.com/wiley-blackwell

The right of the author to be identified as the author of this work has been asserted in accordance with the Copyright, Designs and Patents Act 1988.

Library of Congress Cataloging-in-Publication Data

Complete SAQs for medical finals / Philip Stather . . . [et al.].
p. ; cm.
Includes bibliographical references.
ISBN: 978-1-4051-8928-6
1. Medicine—Examinations, questions, etc. I.   Stather, Philip.
[DNLM: 1. Medicine—Examination Questions. WB 18.2 C738 2010]
R840.C657 2010
610.76—dc22

2009013414

A catalogue record for this book is available from the British Library.

Set in 9.25/12 pt Meridien by Macmillan Publishing Solutions, Chennai, India
Printed and bound in Malaysia by KHL Printing Co Sdn Bhd

1   2010

Contents

Acknowledgements

We'd like to dedicate this book to our families and friends who supported us throughout medical school and finals. We'd also like to thank Ben Townsend, Laura Murphy and all at Wiley-Blackwell for their help throughout the publication process.

Many of the questions in the book are drawn from real clinical scenarios we have experienced on the wards. The names of all individuals have been anonymised. We would like to extend our thanks to all the patients we have seen.

We hope that this book is of help to all students in the critical run-up to exams. Good luck!!!

Preface

When revising for medical finals we were surprised by the lack of a short-answer question book covering all major medical and surgical specialties. On entering the foundation programme we felt that, having just been through the process of finals exams, we were well placed to address this gap in the market.

This book is designed to cover the vast majority of cases which may turn up in finals exams. It includes medicine, surgery and a large variety of specialties, as well as two separate practice papers, with 239 cases in total. It incorporates many (anonymised) cases from our own personal experiences, in order to make the book as realistic as possible.

Please note this book is a revision aid, not an exhaustive textbook, and we would direct you to other Wiley-Blackwell textbooks for any further revision required.

We hope you find this a useful tool for your finals revision, and wish you the best of luck in the future.

Dr P Stather, Dr H Cheshire, Dr J Manton and Dr M Gorecha
May 2009

1 Cardiology

QUESTIONS

1 William, a 66-year-old man, has been brought into the A & E department by ambulance with central chest pain. Paramedics suspect he is having a heart attack, and have given him morphine, oxygen, nitrates and aspirin.

  a What three further questions would you ask him about:

    i) his pain?   *3 marks*

    ii) his other symptoms?   *3 marks*

  b You suspect he is having an acute MI. What is the most important immediate investigation you would request?   *1 mark*

  c You diagnose him with a STEMI. What would be the next step in your management, considering he is currently stable?   *1 mark*

  d Give two further investigations you would request for this man in the long term.   *2 marks*

  e What four medications is he likely to be started on prior to discharge (assuming there are no contraindications)?   *4 marks*

2 Victor, a 72-year-old man, is brought into the A & E department with central crushing chest pain, radiating to his left arm. He looks particularly unwell, is sweating, and has vomited in the ambulance on the way in. His ECG shows no abnormalities.

  a What is the most likely diagnosis?   *1 mark*

  b What further single investigation would you request to confirm this diagnosis?   *1 mark*

  c Give four risk factors for this condition.   *4 marks*

  d Suggest four areas of lifestyle advice you would give this man on discharge.   *4 marks*

Complete SAQs for Medical Finals By P. Stather et al, Published 2010 by Blackwell Publishing, ISBN: 978-1-4501-8928-6.

3 Winifred, an 80-year-old lady, is on her way into A & E under blue lights. She collapsed in the town and an ambulance was called. An ECG showed ST elevation in leads II, III and AVF. Paramedics have given her morphine, oxygen, nitrates and aspirin.

a Where is the location of her infarction? *1 mark*

b Which coronary artery supplies this territory, and is therefore occluded? *1 mark*

c She is given thrombolytic treatment, and a repeat ECG is performed after 1 hour. What are you looking for on this ECG to determine if the thrombolysis has worked? *1 mark*

d If the thrombolysis has been unsuccessful, suggest two treatment options. *2 marks*

e A week later this patient develops mitral regurgitation. Describe the three characteristic findings on auscultation of this murmur. *3 marks*

f Explain the likely cause of this murmur in this patient. *2 marks*

4 Vivian, a 64-year-old lady, who suffers from type 2 diabetes and vascular dementia, has come into A & E with chest pain. You are unable to obtain a history from her, but her husband says the pain began a few hours ago, and she has had it before.

a Name three systems which may cause chest pain, and an example of each. *3 marks*

b Name four investigations you would request immediately for this patient. *4 marks*

c Your tests come back showing that she has had a STEMI. You plan to give thrombolytic agents. Give three contraindications to thrombolysis. *3 marks*

5 Zachary, a 57-year-old man, comes to see you in your GP clinic. He has been having chest pain for the past 2 months, which comes and goes. The pain tends to occur when he walks into town, or up the stairs, and goes after he has rested for a few minutes.

a What is the most likely diagnosis? *1 mark*

b Give three risk factors for this disease. *3 marks*

c Identify three different mechanisms or causes responsible for this condition. *3 marks*

d Give three different types of medication that could be used to help control this condition. *3 marks*

e What are the two surgical options in this case, considering the patient is otherwise healthy? *2 marks*

6 Wilma, a 60-year-old Caucasian lady, has come to see you in the GP surgery. You take her BP, which reads 150/95.

   a What would you do next?   *1 mark*

   b She is diagnosed with essential hypertension and started on medication. Please describe the four steps of the antihypertensive ladder for this patient.   *4 marks*

   c Unfortunately this lady is unable to tolerate an ACE inhibitor as it has been causing her to cough. Explain the biochemical cause of the cough, and what can be done about it.   *2 marks*

   d Give four common causes of secondary hypertension.   *4 marks*

7 Xavier, a 68-year-old man, presents to A & E with collapse. On examination you find an ejection systolic murmur.

   a What diagnosis is this murmur consistent with?   *1 mark*

   b Give two common causes of this condition.   *2 marks*

   c Suggest three symptoms the patient may have because of this.   *3 marks*

   d Give three possible complications of this condition.   *3 marks*

   e What single investigation would you request in order to assess the extent of disease in this valve?   *1 mark*

   f This patient requires replacement of his valve. What different varieties of valves can be used, and what are the pros and cons of each?   *4 marks*

8 Vincent, a 45-year-old man, comes to see you for a routine work physical. You detect no abnormalities, although routine bloods are taken, and his fasting cholesterol is 7.5. You ask him to return to see you in view of this result.

   a Describe two aspects of your initial management of this patient.   *2 marks*

   b He adheres to your initial plan, but it does little to affect his lipid profile. Give two classes of medication you could use in this case.   *2 marks*

   c Suggest two physical features you may elicit in this patient.   *2 marks*

   d Name three other common conditions which may cause raised lipids.   *3 marks*

   e Give three possible common complications of raised cholesterol.   *3 marks*

9 Rhys, a 36-year-old man, who is an IV drug user, is admitted with fever, weight loss and a systolic murmur.

   a What condition are you concerned about in this patient? *1 mark*

   b Give three abnormalities you may detect on examining this patient's hands. *3 marks*

   c What is the most common bacteria causing this condition? *1 mark*

   d What would you do to determine the causative agent? *2 marks*

   e Give three pre-existing conditions that increase the chance of a patient contracting this disease. *3 marks*

   f What single measure may be taken to help prevent those patients at risk of this condition from obtaining it? *1 mark*

10 Morgan, a 32-year-old man, has come in to A & E with chest pain. It is worse when lying flat, and relieved by leaning forwards. He has also noticed difficulty breathing when lying down.

   a What is the medical term for difficulty in breathing on lying down? *1 mark*

   b You suspect pericarditis in this patient. What two abnormalities might you find on auscultation? *2 marks*

   c What would expect to see on an ECG of this patient? *1 mark*

   d What sign may you see on CXR of this patient? *1 mark*

   e Give three possible causes of pericarditis. *3 marks*

   f This patient's condition progresses, and he develops cardiac tamponade. What procedure can be done to relieve the stress on the heart, and name one risk associated with this procedure. *2 marks*

11 Yvonne, a 63-year-old lady, presents with a central chest pain radiating to her back. It feels like a tearing pain, which is spreading down her body. She is sweating profusely and short of breath.

   a What diagnosis are you concerned about in this lady? *1 mark*

   b Suggest two other conditions you would be considering at this stage. *2 marks*

   c Give three aspects of your initial management of this patient. *3 marks*

   d Give two risk factors for this condition. *2 marks*

e What are the two treatment options for this
condition?   *2 marks*

12 Zoe, a 68-year-old lady with a BMI of 35, comes to see you
in the GP surgery. She has been feeling increasingly short of
breath, and has noticed that her ankles have swollen recently.
  a Give the most likely diagnosis.   *1 mark*
  b What three further aspects of the respiratory
      history would you ask about?   *3 marks*
  c Name three blood tests you would do in this
      patient, and why.   *3 marks*
  d What cardiac abnormality may you see on CXR
      in this patient?   *1 mark*
  e What might been seen on ECG in this patient?   *1 mark*
  f What abnormality might be seen on ECHO?   *1 mark*
  g Give two classes of medications that would
      be appropriate in this case.   *2 marks*

13 Douglas, a 70-year-old man, comes into A & E complaining
of palpitations and light-headedness. His pulse is irregularly
irregular, although there is no other abnormality detected on
examination.
  a What is the likely diagnosis?   *1 mark*
  b An ECG is performed. What would you look
      for on the ECG to diagnose this condition?   *1 mark*
  c You decide to try to cardiovert this gentleman.
      Give two different ways of doing this.   *2 marks*
  d Unfortunately the cardioversion is unsuccessful.
      Give three long-term treatments this patient
      may require.   *3 marks*
  e Give three further complications this patient
      is at risk of.   *3 marks*

14 Jenny, a 10-day-old baby, has central cyanosis. She is diagnosed with tetralogy of Fallot.
  a Give two other congenital cardiac causes of
      cyanosis.   *2 marks*
  b What are the four abnormalities present in
      tetralogy of Fallot?   *4 marks*
  c Give three other symptoms of this condition.   *3 marks*
  d What are the three shunts found in the
      circulatory system in utero, which close
      after birth?   *3 marks*

Cardiology

ANSWERS

1 a i) Severity *(1 mark)*, quality *(1 mark)*, radiating   `/3`
       sites (neck, jaw, arm or back) *(1 mark)*
   ii) *(1 mark for each correct answer, maximum 3 marks)*   `/3`
       Associated symptoms – sweating *(1 mark)*,
       pallor *(1 mark)*, SOB *(1 mark)*, cough *(1 mark)*,
       palpitations *(1 mark)*, dizziness *(1 mark)*
  b ECG *(1 mark)*   `/1`
  c Thrombolysis *(1 mark)* – typically with reteplase   `/1`
  d *(1 mark for each correct answer, maximum 3 marks)*   `/2`
     Exercise tolerance test *(1 mark)*
     Angiogram *(1 mark)*
     ECHO *(1 mark)*
  e ACE inhibitor *(1 mark)*   `/4`
     Aspirin 75 mg *(1 mark)*
     Statin *(1 mark)*
     Beta-blocker *(1 mark)*

Summary

Following an MI, NICE guidelines suggest all patients should be advised to undertake physical activity for 20–30 minutes per day, stop smoking and eat a more Mediterranean-style diet. All patients should also ideally be started on an ACE inhibitor, beta blocker, statin and aspirin, and in the case of an NSTEMI then clopidogrel should be added for 12 months. All patients should also be considered for coronary revascularisation.

2 a NSTEMI *(1 mark)*   `/1`
  b Troponin *(1 mark)*   `/1`
  c *(1 mark for each correct answer, maximum 4 marks)*   `/4`
     Smoking *(1 mark)*
     Family history < 50 *(1 mark)*
     Diabetes *(1 mark)*
     Age *(1 mark)*

hypertension *(1 mark)*
Obesity *(1 mark)*
Hypercholesterolaemia *(1 mark)*
Male *(1 mark)*
Ethnicity *(1 mark)*

d *(1 mark for each correct answer, maximum 4 marks)*   /4
Regular attendance with GP to follow up blood
   pressure, cholesterol and diabetes *(1 mark)*
Don't smoke *(1 mark)*
Keep alcohol consumption to a moderate level *(1 mark)*
Eat less fat and more fruit, vegetables and fish – a
   Mediterranean diet *(1 mark)*
Take regular exercise *(1 mark)*
Lose weight *(1 mark)*

Summary
Lifestyle advice and modification of risk factors is important in any condition. Patients acting on such advice can feel they are helping prevent further health problems. However, motivation is often a problem, and some patients require a lot of encouragement.

3 a Inferior *(1 mark)*   /1
  b Right coronary artery *(1 mark)*   /1
  c A decrease in the ST elevation of 50% *(1 mark)*   /1
  d Further thrombolysis *(1 mark)*   /2
    Percutaneous intervention (emergency stenting)
     (1 mark)
  e Pansystolic murmur *(1 mark)*   /3
    Consistent volume *(1 mark)*
    Radiating to the axilla *(1 mark)*
  f Impairment of the blood supply to the area around   /2
    the mitral valve (the valve itself being avascular)
    (1 mark), causing weakening of the papillary muscles
    and rupture of the chordae tendinae *(1 mark)*. In
    some cases the ischaemic cardiac damage can cause
    dilatation of the heart *(1 mark)* leading to
    mitral regurgitation.

Summary
In the majority of patients, the left anterior descending artery supplies the anterior septum, anterior wall, and apex of the heart, the left circumflex artery supplies the lateral wall, and the right coronary artery supplies the posterior, lateral and inferior segments of the heart.

4 a Cardiac – MI, angina, pericarditis, aortic dissection   /3
    (1 mark for the system and 1 example)
    Gastrointestinal – GORD, gastric/peptic ulcer,
    cholecystitis, pancreatitis, strangulated hiatus
    hernia *(1 mark for the system and 1 example)*
    Respiratory – pleurisy, costochondritis, PE,
    pneumothorax, pneumonia *(1 mark for the system
    and 1 example)*
    Musculoskeletal pain – fractured rib, pulled muscle
    (1 mark for the system and 1 example)
b ECG *(1 mark)*   /4
    CXR *(1 mark)*
    Bloods (FBC, U+E, LFT, CRP, glucose, D-dimer)
    (1 mark for any of these, maximum 2 marks)
c *(1 mark for each correct answer, maximum 3 marks)*   /3
    Intracranial haemorrhage *(1 mark)*
    Stroke within the past 3 months *(1 mark)*
    Head injury within the past 3 months *(1 mark)*
    Brain tumours *(1 mark)*
    Pregnancy *(1 mark)*
    Severe hypertension *(1 mark)*
    Major surgery within the past 3 weeks *(1 mark)*
    Internal bleeding within the past 2–4 weeks *(1 mark)*
    Active peptic ulcer disease *(1 mark)*
    Trauma *(1 mark)*

Summary
There are a large number of causes of chest pain, and it is important to be able to distinguish between the different systems causing this, and know what initial investigation must be performed
in these patients. It is imperative that all patients presenting with
chest pain have an ECG done ASAP. A large number of patients
are admitted daily due to chest pain, and discharged 12 hours later
following a negative troponin level and normal CTPA, with a diagnosis of musculoskeletal pain; however, it is important to rule out
more serious pathology.

5 a Angina *(1 mark)*   /1
b *(1 mark for each correct answer, maximum 3 marks)*   /3
    Male *(1 mark)*
    Diabetes *(1 mark)*
    Family history under 50 *(1 mark)*

Hypertension *(1 mark)*
Hypercholesterolaemia *(1 mark)*
Obesity *(1 mark)*
Smoking *(1 mark)*
Ethnicity *(1 mark)*

c *(1 mark for each correct answer, maximum 3 marks)* /3
Decreased coronary perfusion *(1 mark)*
Arrhythmias *(1 mark)*
Anaemia *(1 mark)*
Coronary artery spasm *(1 mark)*
Heart failure *(1 mark)*
Valvular disease *(1 mark)*
Hyperthyroidism *(1 mark)*

d *(1 mark for each correct answer, maximum 3 marks)* /3
GTN or longer acting nitrates *(1 mark)*
Aspirin *(1 mark)*, statins *(1 mark)*
Antihypertensives (beta-blockers, ACEI) *(1 mark)*
Calcium channel blockers *(1 mark)*

e Angioplasty *(1 mark)* /2
CABG *(1 mark)*

Summary

Angina is caused by decreased oxygen supply to the heart. It is a common condition, with the aim of treatment to prevent further deterioration of the condition, and to make the patient symptom free. This is initially done with aspirin, statins, blood pressure control and PRN GTN; however, many patients require further surgical intervention to improve their quality of life.

6 a Obtain repeat BP readings spread over time to /1
determine if she has hypertension. *(1 mark)*
If this remains inconclusive then obtain 24-hour BP.
(1 mark)

b She should be started on either a calcium channel /4
blocker or a diuretic. *(1 mark)*
If this does not control the hypertension then an
ACE inhibitor should be added. *(1 mark)*
The next step is either a calcium channel blocker or
diuretic depending upon your first choice of drug.
(1 mark)
Beta-blockers can be used fourth line. *(1 mark)*

c ACE inhibitors cause a build-up of bradykinin, /2
causing the cough. *(1 mark)*
Her treatment should be changed to an angiotensin
receptor blocker. *(1 mark)*
d *(1 mark for each correct answer, maximum 4 marks)* /4
Glomerular disease *(1 mark)*
Renal artery stenosis *(1 mark)*
COCP *(1 mark)*
Coarctation of the aorta *(1 mark)*
Diabetes *(1 mark)*
Cushing's disease *(1 mark)*
Pregnancy *(1 mark)*
Conn's syndrome *(1 mark)*
Phaeochromocytoma *(1 mark)*

Summary

Essential hypertension accounts for 90–95% of hypertension. The treatment ladder depends on the age and sex of the patient, and any other conditions the patient may have. For young non-black patients the initial treatment is with an ACE inhibitor, however this is second line in those over 55, or any black patient. Secondary causes of hypertension should be looked for through initial screening with blood tests to look for renal disease and diabetes; however, further testing should be reserved for those with resistant hypertension, that is a BP over 150/90 on three antihypertensive agents.

7 a Aortic stenosis *(1 mark)* /1
b *(1 mark for each correct answer, maximum 2 marks)* /2
Rheumatic fever *(1 mark)*
Bicuspid aortic valve *(1 mark)*
Calcification of the aortic valve *(1 mark)*
c *(1 mark for each correct answer, maximum 3 marks)* /3
Fainting *(1 mark)*
Dyspnoea *(1 mark)*
Palpitations *(1 mark)*
Chest pain *(1 mark)*
d *(1 mark for each correct answer, maximum 3 marks)* /3
Left ventricular hypertrophy *(1 mark)*
Left-sided heart failure *(1 mark)*
Arrhythmias *(1 mark)*
Endocarditis *(1 mark)*

e Echocardiogram *(1 mark)*   `/1`
f Metallic valve *(1 mark)* – longer life (20 years)   `/4`
    but requires lifelong warfarin. *(1 mark)*
  Tissue valve graft *(1 mark)* – shorter life (10 years)
    but requires warfarin for only 6 months. *(1 mark)*

Summary

Heart valve replacements have traditionally been performed through open heart surgery; however, newer techniques are now beginning to allow replacement of a valve through percutaneous intervention, which has the added advantage of a much shorter recovery time. The choice between mechanical and artificial valves depends on the co-morbidities and life expectancy of the patient. For example, a young woman who wants children cannot have a metallic valve as she would need to take warfarin, which is teratogenic, whereas a fit 70-year-old man may prefer a metallic valve and to accept the increased risk of bleeds.

8 a Dietary advice (less fat, less alcohol, more fruit   `/2`
      and veg) *(1 mark)*
    Encourage more exercise *(1 mark)*
  b *(1 mark for each correct answer, maximum 2 marks)*   `/2`
    Statins *(1 mark)*
    Fibrates *(1 mark)*
    Bile salt sequestrants *(1 mark)*
    Nicotinic acid *(1 mark)*
  c *(1 mark for each correct answer, maximum 2 marks)*   `/2`
    Xanthelasma *(1 mark)*
    Corneal arcus *(1 mark)*
    Xanthoma *(1 mark)*
  d *(1 mark for each correct answer, maximum 3 marks)*   `/3`
    Diabetes *(1 mark)*
    Hypothyroidism *(1 mark)*
    Cushing's disease *(1 mark)*
    Kidney failure *(1 mark)*
  e *(1 mark for each correct answer, maximum 3 marks)*   `/3`
    Atherosclerosis *(1 mark)*
    Coronary artery disease *(1 mark)*
    Stroke *(1 mark)*
    MI *(1 mark)*
    Peripheral vascular disease *(1 mark)*

Summary

Treatment of hypercholesterolaemia has been shown to significantly reduce morbidity and mortality across populations. Treatment should be initiated in all patients with a raised cholesterol level, and statins are used for secondary prevention in patients following MI, angina, stroke, TIA, or peripheral arterial disease.

9 a Subacute bacterial endocarditis *(1 mark)* `/1`
   b *(1 mark for each correct answer, maximum 3 marks)* `/3`
     Janeway lesions *(1 mark)*
     Osler nodes *(1 mark)*
     Splinting haemorrhages *(1 mark)*
     Septic emboli/gangrene *(1 mark)*
     Clubbing *(1 mark)*
   c *Streptococcus viridans (1 mark)* `/1`
   d Blood cultures *(1 mark)* taken from 3 different `/2`
     sites, separated over time *(1 mark)*
   e *(1 mark for each correct answer, maximum 3 marks)* `/3`
     Congenital heart disease *(1 mark)*
     Rheumatic heart disease *(1 mark)*
     Cardiac valve anomalies *(1 mark)*
     Artificial heart valves *(1 mark)*
   f Prophylactic antibiotics before invasive procedures `/1`
     (1 mark)

Summary

Infective endocarditis is an infection involving the endocardial surface of the heart, which causes valvular insufficiency, causing congestive heart failure, and possibly abscesses on the myocardium. Emboli from the valve, which may be infective, along with immune reactions, cause the variety of signs and symptoms of the condition. Infective endocarditis should be suspected in any patient with a fever and newly diagnosed heart murmur.

10 a Orthopnoea *(1 mark)* `/1`
   b Muffled heart sounds *(1 mark)* `/2`
     Pericardial rub *(1 mark)*
   c Saddle-shaped ST segment throughout the `/1`
     majority of the leads *(1 mark)*
   d Globular heart *(1 mark)* `/1`
   e *(1 mark for each correct answer, maximum 3 marks)* `/3`

Infection *(1 mark)*
Autoimmune disorders *(1 mark)*
Rheumatic fever *(1 mark)*
TB *(1 mark)*
Cancer *(1 mark)*
Leukaemia *(1 mark)*
Renal failure *(1 mark)*
HIV *(1 mark)*
Hypothyroidism *(1 mark)*

f Pericardiocentesis *(1 mark)* /2
   Risks of puncturing the myocardium or a coronary
   artery, MI, needle induced arrhythmias,
   pneumopericardium, infection, and accidental
   puncture of other organs *(1 mark for any of these
   examples)*

Summary
Pericarditis may be idiopathic, although is caused by several conditions, such as infections, autoimmune conditions, MI (Dressler's syndrome), trauma to the heart, malignancy, and as a side effect of medications. Patients typically present with chest pain radiating to the back, which is relieved by sitting forward, and exacerbated by lying down. They may also have a cough, fever and fatigue.

11 a Aortic dissection *(1 mark)* /1
   b *(1 mark for each correct answer, maximum 2 marks)* /2
      MI *(1 mark)*
      Pericarditis *(1 mark)*
      Musculoskeletal pain *(1 mark)*
      Aortic aneurysm *(1 mark)*
   c *(1 mark for each correct answer, maximum 3 marks)* /3
      ABC *(1 mark)*
      Check blood pressure on both arms *(1 mark)*
      Request CT scan if unsure of the diagnosis and
         the patient is stable *(1 mark)*
      Refer to surgeons urgently *(1 mark)*
   d *(1 mark for each correct answer, maximum 2 marks)* /2
      Atherosclerosis *(1 mark)*
      Hypertension *(1 mark)*
      Traumatic injury *(1 mark)*
      Connective tissue disorders *(1 mark)*

e Medical management – pain relief and ensuring   /2
  the blood pressure is stable *(1 mark)*
  Surgical repair or replacement of the aorta *(1 mark)*

Summary
Aortic dissection resulting in rupture has an 80% mortality rate, with the majority of patients not making it into hospital. If you suspect a patient has a dissection you must phone the surgical registrar on call immediately. Take blood samples from the patient including cross match of at least 6 units, and do not give any fluids, as this will increase their BP and increase the risk of further haemorrhage. They must be operated on ASAP, then they can be fluid resuscitated.

12 a Heart failure *(1 mark)*   /1
  b *(1 mark for each correct answer, maximum 3 marks)*   /3
   Smoking *(1 mark)*
   Orthopnoea *(1 mark)*
   Paroxysmal nocturnal dyspnoea *(1 mark)*
   Cough *(1 mark)*
   Sputum production *(1 mark)*
  c FBC – look for anaemia *(1 mark)*   /3
   U+E – assess renal function, which may affect fluid
    balance *(1 mark)*
   LFT – fluid overload can cause congestion of the liver,
    and a low albumin can cause fluid overload *(1 mark)*
  d Cardiomegaly (cardiothoracic ratio >50%) *(1 mark)*   /1
  e Left ventricular hypertrophy (S in V1 + R in V5   /1
   or V6 >35mm) *(1 mark)*
  f Decreased ejection fraction (<40%) *(1 mark)*   /1
  g *(1 mark for each correct answer, maximum 2 marks)*   /2
   Diuretics *(1 mark)*
   ACE inhibitors *(1 mark)*
   Beta-blockers *(1 mark)*

Summary
Congestive cardiac failure is an impairment of the heart's ability to pump blood around the body, causing fluid overload. The NYHA classification of heart failure gives four categories of severity of heart failure depending on the activity of the patient:
  Class I – no limitation and asymptomatic
  Class II – Slight, mild limitation of activity, although the patient
   is comfortable at rest

Class III – Marked limitation of any activity, with the patient only comfortable at rest
Class IV – Discomfort and symptoms occur with any activity and at rest.

13 a Atrial fibrillation *(1 mark)*　　　　　　　　　　　　　　　　`/1`
   b Absence of 'p' waves *(1 mark)*　　　　　　　　　　　　　　`/1`
   c Electrical *(1 mark)*　　　　　　　　　　　　　　　　　　　`/2`
       Medical (amiodarone, sotalol, or flecainide) *(1 mark)*
   d Digoxin *(1 mark)*　　　　　　　　　　　　　　　　　　　　`/3`
       Beta-blockers *(1 mark)*
       Warfarin *(1 mark)*
   e *(1 mark for each correct answer, maximum 3 marks)*　　　`/3`
       PE *(1 mark)*
       Stroke *(1 mark)*
       Transient ischaemic attack *(1 mark)*
       Collapse *(1 mark)*

Summary

Atrial fibrillation can occur due to a variety of cardiac causes, such as coronary artery disease, mitral stenosis, mitral regurgitation, HOCM, pericarditis, congenital heart disease, and previous cardiac surgery, as well as hypertension, lung disease, alcohol, hyperthyroidism and carbon monoxide poisoning. Treatment involves rate control to try to revert the patient back into sinus rhythm, and anticoagulation, in order to prevent thrombo-embolic events.

14 a *(1 mark for each correct answer, maximum 2 marks)*　　　`/2`
       Transposition of the great arteries *(1 mark)*
       Total anomalous pulmonary venous return *(1 mark)*
       Truncus arteriosus *(1 mark)*, tricuspid atresia *(1 mark)*
       Hypoplastic left heart syndrome *(1 mark)*
   b Ventricular septal defect *(1 mark)*　　　　　　　　　　　`/4`
       Pulmonary stenosis *(1 mark)*
       Over-riding aorta *(1 mark)*
       Right ventricular hypertrophy *(1 mark)*
   c *(1 mark for each correct answer, maximum 3 marks)*　　　`/3`
       Difficulty feeding *(1 mark)*
       Developmental delay *(1 mark)*
       Poor weight gain *(1 mark)*
       Clubbing *(1 mark)*
       Sudden death *(1 mark)*

d Ductus arteriosus *(1 mark)*   /3

Ductus venosus *(1 mark)*

Foramen ovale *(1 mark)*

Summary

The foramen ovale may be kept patent for a short period of time by the use of prostin. This is done with patients where the blood flow to the lungs from the right ventricle is inadequate to maintain sufficient oxygenation for life. These patients may then have their congenital defects corrected, or a shunt put in place from a branch of the aorta to the pulmonary artery.

2 Respiratory Medicine

QUESTIONS

1 Andrew, a 14-year-old asthmatic schoolboy, is brought to see you by his mum. She reports that today he has been having difficulty in breathing, with a dry cough, wheezing and chest tightness.
  a Give four differential diagnoses of acute dyspnoea.   *4 marks*
  b Explain the pathophysiology behind asthma.   *3 marks*
  c Give three features of life-threatening asthma.   *3 marks*
  d Give four aspects of the acute management of severe asthma.   *4 marks*

2 Joyce, an 89-year-old lady in a residential home, presents with a 5-day history of dyspnoea, productive cough, fever and chest pain. On examination she is pyrexial and tachycardic with left basal crepitations. Her oxygen saturations are 94% on air.
  a State the likely diagnosis.   *1 mark*
  b Name two risk factors for this condition in any patient.   *2 marks*
  c Name two investigations you would request, and the abnormality likely to be seen.   *2 marks*
  d Name the three likely causative organisms responsible for this disease.   *3 marks*
  e Explain what CURB-65 stands for and the values used.   *2 marks*
  f State one complication of this condition.   *1 mark*

3 Anita, a 17-year-old A-level student, attends your surgery complaining that her blue inhaler is not helping her asthma and she is often breathless. You notice she has dry skin on both hands and after questioning she reveals her mum and sister both suffer from similar conditions.

Complete SAQs for Medical Finals By P. Stather et al, Published 2010 by Blackwell Publishing, ISBN: 978-1-4501-8928-6.

a Name two other conditions often associated with
   asthma.   *2 marks*
b You explain to her about asthma triggers; please
   identify four common triggers.   *4 marks*
c You manage her asthma according to BTS
   guidelines, what are the five steps of management?   *5 marks*
d What two strategies would you use to prevent relapse?   *2 marks*
e What is atopy?   *1 mark*

4 Judith, a 66-year-old lifelong smoker, has always had breathing
   problems, but is now increasingly dyspnoeic. She has a chronic
   productive cough but says her sputum colour has changed and
   increased in volume. On examination she is using her accessory muscles of respiration, has a hyperexpanded chest and an
   audible wheeze.

a What are the three pathological changes in bronchitis?   *3 marks*
b Name one accessory muscle of respiration   *1 mark*
c Apart from blood tests, give two simple
   investigations you would request.   *2 marks*
d What does this ABG show?   *2 marks*

   pH   7.30   (7.35–7.45)
   pO_2 7.4   (11–13)
   pCO_2 10.2   (4.5–6)
   Bicarb   22   (21–28)
   BE   2   (+/–2)

e It was suspected that this exacerbation was caused
   by a chest infection. Outline four aspects of your
   management.   *4 marks*

5 Craig, a 46-year-old male with peripheral vascular disease, had
   an above-knee amputation 14 days ago. He is now complaining
   of sudden-onset shortness of breath and haemoptysis. On examination he is breathless, tachypnoeic, tachycardic and hypoxic.

a What diagnosis do you suspect?   *1 mark*
b Name three investigations you would request.   *3 marks*
c This is the ABG result on 5 L of oxygen – please
   interpret the result.   *2 marks*

   pH   7.47   (7.35–7.45)
   pO_2 8.2   (11–13)
   pCO_2 3.4   (4.5–6)
   Bicarb   22   (21–28)
   BE   2   (+/–2)

   d Give six risk factors for a thromboembolism.   *3 marks*
   e What two medications would you initiate?   *2 marks*

6 Paula, a 30-year-old woman who has never smoked, presents to you with shortness of breath. She tells you that she was diagnosed with bronchiectasis 3 years ago and is frequently hospitalised due to chest infections.

   a What is the pathology of bronchiectasis?   *2 marks*
   b Give three clinical features of bronchiectasis.   *3 marks*
   c Name four causes of bronchiectasis.   *4 marks*
   d Other than a CXR, what three investigations
      would you request?   *3 marks*

7 Sagheer, a 38-year-old Asian male, comes to see you in your surgery. He has recently returned from visiting relatives in India and is concerned because he has found out that one of the relatives he stayed with has just been diagnosed with tuberculosis.

   a What is the causative organism?   *1 mark*
   b Give three further symptoms or signs you would
      ask about to clarify your diagnosis.   *3 marks*
   c Apart from a CXR, what three investigations
      would you request?   *3 marks*
   d Give two abnormalities you may see on Sagheer's
      chest x-ray.   *2 marks*
   e Name the four drugs used in the treatment
      of tuberculosis and an associated side effect
      of each.   *4 marks*

8 Tallulah, a 45-year-old lady who recently moved to the UK from the Bahamas, presents with a 4-month history of dyspnoea, decreased exercise tolerance, mild fever and arthralgia. Investigations are consistent with a diagnosis of sarcoidosis.

   a Name two differential diagnoses.   *2 marks*
   b Other than the symptoms mentioned in Tallulah's
      history give four extrapulmonary features of this
      condition.   *4 marks*
   c What four investigations may have been
      requested prior to confirmation of
      sarcoidosis?   *4 marks*
   d What treatment would you initiate?   *1 mark*

9 Arthur, a 54-year-old farmer, presents with acute dyspnoea, fever and malaise which began shortly after he cleaned his hay loft out. On examination he is tachypnoeic with wheezing and coarse end-inspiratory crackles.

a What diagnosis do you suspect?   *1 mark*

b Give four investigations you would request.   *4 marks*

c You start him on steroids. Name four side-effects of long-term steroid use.   *4 marks*

d Name two other occupations/hobbies which predispose to developing this condition.   *2 marks*

10 Sid, a 76-year-old male who used to work in the coal mines, presents with increasing dyspnoea and a cough productive of black sputum. You notice he has clubbing.

a What is the likely diagnosis?   *1 mark*

b What is the underlying pathophysiology?   *3 marks*

c What would you look for on a chest x ray?   *1 mark*

d Identify two non-respiratory systems where clubbing is seen, and give two examples of each.   *3 marks*

e Asbestos is another problematic compound; give three lung diseases it may cause.   *3 marks*

11 Paul, an 83-year-old lifelong smoker presents with a cough of a few months' duration. He has recently noticed haemoptysis, dyspnoea and weight loss. You also notice that his voice is hoarse today and his left eyelid appears to be drooping.

a What is the likely diagnosis and syndrome it is causing?   *2 mark*

b Give two histological types of lung carcinoma.   *2 marks*

c Apart from blood tests give three investigations you would perform.   *3 marks*

d Give four extra-pulmonary non-metastatic manifestations of bronchial carcinoma.   *4 marks*

e Give two of the treatment options available.   *2 marks*

12 Claire, 47, presents with a decreasing exercise tolerance and sharp chest pain on deep inspiration. On examination there is tracheal shift, absent breath sounds and dullness to percussion at the left base.

a What is the diagnosis?   *1 mark*

b Give the two different types of fluid according to the protein content, and two examples of each cause.   *6 marks*

  c You take a pleural fluid aspirate. What four
    tests will you perform on the fluid?   *4 marks*
  d How could you manage the effusion?   *1 mark*

13 Sarah, a 17-year-old girl, is brought into A & E after a road traffic
collision. She was initially feeling well but is now suddenly very
short of breath with chest pains. On examination she is tachycardic, tachypnoeic and cyanotic with absent breath sounds on
the left side.

  a What is the immediate treatment and describe
    the anatomical landmarks you would use.   *3 marks*
  b Give five causes of a pneumothorax.   *5 marks*
  c Give three chest x-ray findings in a patient with
    a simple pneumothorax.   *3 marks*
  d Sarah presents twice in the next 3 months with
    recurrent pneumothoraces.
    What two pieces of advice would you give her?   *2 marks*
    What would the best treatment option be now?   *1 mark*

Respiratory Medicine
ANSWERS

1 a *(1 mark for each correct answer, maximum 4 marks)*   `/4`
Asthma *(1 mark)*
Pneumothorax *(1 mark)*
Pneumonia *(1 mark)*
Pulmonary embolism *(1 mark)*
mi *(1 mark)*
Heart failure *(1 mark)*
Pulmonary oedema *(1 mark)*
copd (exacerbation) *(1 mark)*

b Bronchial hypersensitivity causes bronchial   `/3`
inflammation *(1 mark)* and bronchial constriction
(1 mark), with excess mucus production *(1 mark)*

c *(1 mark for each correct answer, maximum 3 marks)*   `/3`
PEFR <33% predicted *(1 mark)*
SATs <92% *(1 mark)*
pO_2 <8 *(1 mark)*
Silent chest *(1 mark)*
Cyanosis *(1 mark)*
Poor respiratory effort *(1 mark)*
Exhaustion *(1 mark)*
Confusion *(1 mark)*
Bradycardia *(1 mark)*

d *(1 mark for each correct answer, maximum 4 marks)*   `/4`
Admit the patient *(1 mark)*
High flow oxygen *(1 mark)*
Nebulised salbutamol *(1 mark)*
IV hydrocortisone *(1 mark)*
Nebulised ipatropium bromide *(1 mark)*
IV magnesium sulphate infusion *(1 mark)*
Senior support and contact ITU if appropriate *(1 mark)*

Summary
Patients with severe asthma typically present with acute SOB and respiratory distress. Severe asthma can potentially be life threatening,

and treatment with salbutamol nebulisers, hydrocortisone and ipra-tropium should be instigated immediately. Physiologically asthma is a chronic inflammatory disease of the airways with three character-istic features: reversible airflow limitation, bronchial inflammation and hyper-responsiveness of the airways. The associated pathologi-cal changes involve eosinophils, T lymphocytes and mast cells caus-ing airway oedema and smooth muscle hypertrophy.

2 a Community acquired pneumonia *(1 mark)* ☐ /1
  b *(1 mark for each correct answer, maximum 2 marks)* ☐ /2
    Elderly *(1 mark)*
    Smoking *(1 mark)*
    Underlying respiratory disease *(1 mark)*
    Immunosuppression *(1 mark)*
  c *(1 mark for each correct answer, maximum 2 marks)* ☐ /2
    WCC raised *(1 mark)*
    CRP raised *(1 mark)*
    CXR showing consolidation *(1 mark)*
    ABG showing hypoxia *(1 mark)*
  d *Streptococcus pneumoniae (1 mark)* ☐ /3
    Haemophilus influenzae (1 mark)
    Mycoplasma pneumoniae (1 mark)
  e Confusion of new onset *(1 mark)* ☐ /2
    Urea >7 *(1 mark)*
    RR >30 *(1 mark)*
    Systolic BP <90 *(1 mark)*
    Age over 65 *(1 mark)*
  f *(1 mark for each correct answer, maximum 1 mark)* ☐ /1
    Lung abscess *(1 mark)*
    Septicaemia *(1 mark)*
    Respiratory failure *(1 mark)*
    Empyema *(1 mark)*
    Death *(1 mark)*

Summary
Patients with pneumonia typically present with pyrexia and a produc-tive cough. There will be crepitations on examination. Community acquired pneumonia is typically treated with amoxicillin, and atypi-cal pneumonia with erythromycin. The CURB65 score is an impor-tant step in determining the severity of pneumonia. Depending upon severity patients are managed using oral or intravenous antibiotics,

fluids and chest physiotherapy. Choice of antibiotics is determined by local policy and any sputum cultures and sensitivities available.

3 a *(1 mark for each correct answer, maximum 2 marks)* `/2`
Eczema *(1 mark)*
Allergic rhinitis *(1 mark)*
Peanut/food allergies *(1 mark)*
Hay fever *(1 mark)*
b *(1 mark for each correct answer, maximum 4 marks)* `/4`
Pollen *(1 mark)*
Dust mite *(1 mark)*
Animals *(1 mark)*
Aerosols *(1 mark)*
Exercise *(1 mark)*
Infection *(1 mark)*
Chemicals *(1 mark)*
Smoking *(1 mark)*
c Step 1 – inhaled short-acting beta-2 agonist *(1 mark)* `/5`
Step 2 – add inhaled steroid *(1 mark)*
Step 3 – add long-acting beta-2 agonist *(1 mark)*
Step 4 – increased inhaled steroid and leukotriene
  receptor antagonist, slow-release theophylline *(1 mark)*
Step 5 – daily oral steroid tablets *(1 mark)*
d *(1 mark for each correct answer, maximum 2 marks)* `/2`
Good inhaler technique *(1 mark)*
Check medication compliance *(1 mark)*
Avoidance of triggers *(1 mark)*
Encourage exercise to increase lung capacity
  (1 mark)
e A group of disorders that often runs in families `/1`
caused by an IgE related hypersensitivity reaction.
(1 mark)

Summary

Patients tend to present with wheezing, shortness of breath and chest tightness which fluctuates. Treatment is with salbutamol inhalers initially and further treatments are added as required based on the BTS guidelines. Atopy commonly runs in families and may be triggered by contact with any number of common household allergens such as dust, pets and aerosols. Management of asthmatics can be difficult, especially if their compliance is poor or they suffer frequent exacerbations, but guidance is available from the British Thoracic Society.

4 a Narrowed airways *(1 mark)*   □ /3
Reduced airflow *(1 mark)*
Hypertrophy and hyperplasia of mucus glands *(1 mark)*
  b *(1 mark for each correct answer, maximum 1 mark)*   □ /1
Sternocleidomastoid *(1 mark)*
Abdominal muscles *(1 mark)*
Intercostal muscles *(1 mark)*
  c *(1 mark for each correct answer, maximum 2 marks)*   □ /2
Spirometry *(1 mark)*
CXR *(1 mark)*
Sputum culture *(1 mark)*
  d Respiratory *(1 mark)* acidosis *(1 mark)*   □ /2
(type 2 respiratory failure)
  e *(1 mark for each correct answer, maximum 4 marks)*   □ /4
Oxygen carefully titrated according to serial ABGs
    (1 mark)
Nebulised salbutamol *(1 mark)*
Cortiocosteroids *(1 mark)*
Antibiotics according to local protocol *(1 mark)*
Consider ventilatory support, e.g. NIV *(1 mark)*

Summary

COPD tends to occur in those people with a significant smoking history and they tend to develop symptoms of shortness of breath, regular productive cough and poor exercise tolerance. These patients can present with severe exacerbations often preceded by infections or extremes of weather and often develop respiratory failure. It is also seen in some genetic disorders (alpha-1 antitrypsin deficiency) and after occupational exposure to certain substances. Spirometry shows an obstructive pattern with an FEV1/FVC ratio of less than 70% predicted.

5 a Pulmonary embolism *(1 mark)*   □ /1
  b *(1 mark for each correct answer, maximum 3 marks)*   □ /3
ABG – hypoxia/respiratory alkalosis *(1 mark)*
ECG – tachycardia, S1 Q3 T3 *(1 mark)*
CXR – wedge-shaped infarct, consolidation,
    effusion *(1 mark)*
CTPA – filling defects *(1 mark)*
Clotting screen *(1 mark)*

   c Respiratory *(1 mark)* alkalosis *(1 mark)* with hypoxia   `/2`
   d *(½ mark for each correct answer, maximum 3 marks)*   `/3`
      Major surgery within the last 3 months *(½ mark)*
      Age *(½ mark)*
      Major fracture *(½ mark)*
      Obesity *(½ mark)*
      Cancer *(½ mark)*
      Varicose veins *(½ mark)*
      Pregnancy *(½ mark)*
      Thrombophilia *(½ mark)*
      Immobility, e.g. prolonged bed rest, long-haul
        flight *(½ mark)*
      Protein c/s deficiency *(½ mark)*
      Antiphospholipid syndrome *(½ mark)*
      Antithrombin deficiency *(½ mark)*
   e Enoxaparin (1.5 mg/kg) *(1 mark)*   `/2`
      Warfarin *(1 mark)*

Summary
Patients tend to present with sudden onset of shortness of breath, pleuritic chest pain, haemoptysis and tachycardia. It is important to make the diagnosis as otherwise pulmonary embolism can be fatal. A CTPA should be done to establish a diagnosis and treatment is initiated if there is any clinical suspicion. A pulmonary embolism occurs when a thrombus from the systemic circulation becomes dislodged and occludes one of the pulmonary arteries. This causes a ventilation perfusion mismatch. Blood gases demonstrate hypoxia.

6 a *(1 mark for each correct answer, maximum 2 marks)*   `/2`
      Bronchi permanently dilated *(1 mark)*
      Impaired mucus clearance *(1 mark)*
      Bacterial infection causes damage *(1 mark)*
   b *(1 mark for each correct answer, maximum 3 marks)*   `/3`
      Sputum production *(1 mark)*
      Recurrent pneumonia *(1 mark)*
      Halitosis *(1 mark)*
      Clubbing *(1 mark)*
      Coarse crepitations *(1 mark)*
      Dyspnoea *(1 mark)*, haemoptysis *(1 mark)*
   c Idiopathic *(1 mark)*   `/4`
      Infection – measles, whooping cough, pertussis
        (1 mark)

Obstruction – foreign body, tumour *(1 mark)*
Congenital – cystic fibrosis, Kartagener's syndrome
(1 mark)
d HRCT *(1 mark)*   ⬛ /3
Sputum culture *(1 mark)*
Inflammatory markers *(1 mark)*

Summary
Patients with bronchiectasis have often suffered from a respiratory illness in childhood which has led to scarring of the lungs, giving rise to bronchiectasis in adulthood. In bronchiectasis, the airway passages become abnormally dilated with associated inflammation and thickening. This causes irreversible damage and impairs the mucociliary escalator causing increased susceptibility to bacterial infections, creating a vicious cycle of further infection and damage. As a result patients present with a chronic cough productive of copious amounts of white sputum.

7 a *Mycobacterium tuberculosis (1 mark)*   ⬛ /1
   b *(1 mark for each correct answer, maximum 3 marks)*   ⬛ /3
   Cough *(1 mark)*
   Haemoptysis *(1 mark)*
   Malaise *(1 mark)*
   Lethargy *(1 mark)*
   Weight loss *(1 mark)*
   Night sweats *(1 mark)*
   Fever *(1 mark)*
   Anorexia *(1 mark)*
   Lymphadenopathy *(1 mark)*
   c *(1 mark for each correct answer, maximum 3 marks)*   ⬛ /3
   Ziehl-Nielsen sputum stain for AAFB *(1 mark)*
   Sputum culture *(1 mark)*
   Bronchoscopy *(1 mark)*
   Mantoux test *(1 mark)*
   Biopsy + histology *(1 mark)*
   CT scan *(1 mark)*
   d *(1 mark for each correct answer, maximum 2 marks)*   ⬛ /2
   Consolidation *(1 mark)*
   Cavitation *(1 mark)*
   Calcification *(1 mark)*
   Fibrosis *(1 mark)*
   Loss of lung volume *(1 mark)*
   Pleural effusion *(1 mark)*

   e Rifampicin – orange urine, hepatitis, gastrointestinal   `/4`
      symptoms, flu-like symptoms *(1 mark)*
      Isoniazid – polyneuropathy, psychotic episodes,
      vertigo, nausea and vomiting *(1 mark)*
      Pyrazinamide – gout, rash, arthralgia, hepatotoxicity
      (1 mark)
      Ethambutol – optic retrobulbar neuritis *(1 mark)*

Summary

Tuberculosis is a disease characterised by caseating granulomas and the patient tends to present with cough, haemoptysis, weight loss and fever and it is important to take a detailed travel and contact history. The diagnosis is made on bronchial biopsies and treatment involves an intensive regime of antibiotics for many months. Tuberculosis is an important diagnosis to be aware of in view of increased global travel. It is a notifiable disease in Britain and any patient with suspected tuberculosis should be barrier nursed in isolation.

8 a *(1 mark for each correct answer, maximum 2 marks)*   `/2`
      Lymphoma *(1 mark)*
      Tuberculosis *(1 mark)*
      Carcinoma of bronchus *(1 mark)*
      Systemic lupus erythematosus *(1 mark)*
      Beryllium poisoning *(1 mark)*
   b *(1 mark for each correct answer, maximum 4 marks)*   `/4`
      Skin – erythema nodosum, lupus pernio *(1 mark)*
      Eye – anterior uveitis, conjunctivitis *(1 mark)*
      Bone – bone cysts *(1 mark)*
      Metabolic – hypercalcaemia *(1 mark)*
      Liver – hepatosplenomegaly *(1 mark)*
      Nervous system – cranial nerve palsy *(1 mark)*
      Heart – arrhythmias, cardiomyopathy *(1 mark)*
   c *(1 mark for each correct answer, maximum 4 marks)*   `/4`
      Calcium levels *(1 mark)*
      ESR *(1 mark)*
      FBC *(1 mark)*
      LFTs *(1 mark)*
      CXR *(1 mark)*
      Immunoglobulins *(1 mark)*
      Broncho-alveolar lavage *(1 mark)*
      Serum ACE *(1 mark)*
   d Steroids *(1 mark)* and other immunosuppressive   `/1`
      agents.

Summary

Sarcoidosis is a non-caseating granulomatous disease with multi-system involvement characteristically presenting with fever, bilateral hilar lymphadenopathy, erythema nodosum and arthralgia, which can affect all joints of the body. Treatment is with steroids and other immunosuppressive drugs.

9 a Extrinsic allergic alveolitis (farmer's lung) *(1 mark)*   `/1`

   b *(1 mark for each correct answer, maximum 4 marks)*   `/4`
   CXR *(1 mark)*
   Bloods (FBC, U+E, CRP) *(maximum 1 mark)*
   Spirometry *(1 mark)*
   Precipitating antibodies *(1 mark)*
   Bronchoalveolar lavage *(1 mark)*

   c *(1 mark for each correct answer, maximum 4 marks)*   `/4`
   Cataracts *(1 mark)*
   Bruising *(1 mark)*
   Increased abdominal fat *(1 mark)*
   Muscle wasting *(1 mark)*
   Buffalo hump *(1 mark)*
   Hypertension *(1 mark)*
   Osteoporosis *(1 mark)*
   Impotence *(1 mark)*
   Impaired glucose tolerance *(1 mark)*

   d Bird-fancier's lung – proteins in bird faeces *(1 mark)*   `/2`
   Malt worker's lung – *Aspergillus clavatus (1 mark)*

Summary

Patients with extrinsic allergic alveolitis present with dyspnoea, dry cough, fever, and arthralgia. It occurs where long term exposure to an antigen causes the body to produce immunoglobins against the antigen. Upon re-exposure this leads to an inflammatory reaction with granulomas forming around the antigens. If exposure persists the inflammatory response will eventually lead to the development of pulmonary fibrosis.

10 a Coal worker's pneumoconiosis *(1 mark)*   `/1`

   b *(1 mark for each correct answer, maximum 3 marks)*   `/3`
   Small inorganic dust particles *(1 mark)* not
      cleared by the mucociliary system *(1 mark)*,
      reach acinus *(1 mark)*, damage macrophages
      (1 mark), causing inflammation and fibrosis
      (1 mark)

c Pulmonary nodules *(1 mark)*   /1

d Cardiac – cyanotic heart disease, infective   /4
   endocarditis *(1 mark)*
   Gastrointestinal – cirrhosis, inflammatory bowel
      disease *(1 mark)*

e Mesothelioma *(1 mark)*   /3
   Asbestosis *(1 mark)*
   Lung cancer *(1 mark)*

Summary

Exposure to certain agents at work can result in the development of certain lung conditions with examples including bronchitis, fibrosis and malignancy. Coal worker's pneumoconiosis involves microscopic dust particles which become trapped within the small airway passages. This is the commonest dust disease in the UK and there may be compensation available for sufferers.

11 a Pancoast tumour *(1 mark)*   /2
   Horner's syndrome *(1 mark)*

   b *(1 mark for each correct answer, maximum*   /2
      2 marks)
   Squamous *(1 mark)*
   Large cell *(1 mark)*
   Adenocarcinoma *(1 mark)*
   Alveolar cell *(1 mark)*
   Small cell *(1 mark)*

   c *(1 mark for each correct answer, maximum 3 marks)*   /3
   Sputum for cytology *(1 mark)*
   Staging CT *(1 mark)*
   Bronchoscopy *(1 mark)*
   Biopsy *(1 mark)*

   d *(1 mark for each correct answer, maximum 4 marks)*   /4
   Endocrine – ACTH, ADH *(1 mark)*
   Neurological – polyneuropathies *(1 mark)*
   Haematological – anaemia, disseminated
      intravascular coagulation *(1 mark)*
   Skeletal – clubbing *(1 mark)*
   Skin – acanthosis nigricas *(1 mark)*

   e *(1 mark for each correct answer, maximum*   /2
      2 marks)
   Surgery *(1 mark)*
   Radiotherapy *(1 mark)*
   Chemotherapy *(1 mark)*

Summary

Patients with lung cancer may present with chronic SOB, weight loss and haemoptysis, although could present following an unresolving chest infection, or on routine CXR. CT chest abdomen and pelvis is done for staging of the cancer, and biopsy may be required prior to initiating treatment.

Horner's syndrome is characterised by a unilateral meiosis, ptosis and enophthalmos associated with damage to the sympathetic pathway. There are many different causes of Horner's syndrome including cerebral infarct, cord tumour, cervical rib and carotid artery dissection.

12 a Pleural effusion *(1 mark)*   `/1`

   b *(1 mark for each protein level, 2 marks for any 2 causes*   `/6`
      of transudate and 2 marks for any 2 causes of exudate,
      maximum 6 marks)
      Transudate (Protein <30 g/L): cardiac failure,
        hypothyroid, nephrotic syndrome, Meig's
        syndome, renal failure
      Exudate (protein >30 g/L): pneumonia, lung
        carcinoma, pulmonary infarct, tuberculosis,
        connective tissue disease

   c *(1 mark for each correct answer, maximum 3 marks)*   `/4`
      Protein count *(1 mark)*
      LDH *(1 mark)*
      Bacterial culture and sensitivity *(1 mark)*
      Cytology *(1 mark)*
      Cell count *(1 mark)*
      Glucose *(1 mark)*

   d Chest drain *(1 mark)*   `/1`

Summary

A pleural effusion is due to the accumulation of fluid in the pleural space and is detected on chest x-ray when more than 300 ml is present. Treatment is by insertion of a chest drain with fluid sent for cytology, microbiology, glucose, LDH, protein levels and pH. With recurrent pleural effusions, pleurodesis may be required. This is successful in 60–70% of cases.

13 a Needle thoracocentesis *(1 mark)*   `/3`
      Second intercostal space *(1 mark)*
      Mid clavicular line *(1 mark)*

b *(1 mark for each correct answer, maximum*   /5
  5 marks)
Trauma *(1 mark)*
Barotrauma *(1 mark)*
Asthma *(1 mark)*
COPD *(1 mark)*
Tuberculosis *(1 mark)*
Pneumonia *(1 mark)*
Lung abscess *(1 mark)*
Lung carcinoma *(1 mark)*
Cystic fibrosis *(1 mark)*
Sarcoidosis *(1 mark)*
Connective tissue disorders, e.g. Ehlers-Danlos
  syndrome, Marfan's syndrome *(1 mark)*
Iatrogenic – CVP line insertion, pleural aspiration
  or biopsy, percutaneous liver biopsy, positive
  pressure ventilation, tracheostomy insertion,
  OGD, CPR *(1 mark)*
Idiopathic *(1 mark)*
c *(1 mark for each correct answer, maximum 3 marks)*   /3
Tracheal and midline shift *(1 mark)*
Decreased lung markings *(1 mark)*
Raised hemidiaphragm *(1 mark)*
Unequal chest expansion *(1 mark)*
d Advise to refrain from diving *(1 mark)*   /3
Advise to refrain from flying for 1 week
  following resolution on CXR if spontaneous,
  or 2 weeks if traumatic according to BTS
  guidelines *(1 mark)*
Should be offered pleurodesis *(1 mark)*

Summary

Pneumothoraces may occur spontaneously in apparently healthy young males who are tall and thin. Smokers have a higher chance of recurrence than non-smokers and, as with all respiratory patients should be encouraged to quit. Patients typically present with sudden-onset shortness of breath with chest pain, and will have hyper-resonance on that side with decreased air entry, and possibly tracheal deviation.

3 Gastroenterology

QUESTIONS

1 You're the SHO working in A & E, and are presented with James (a 43-year-old male) and his wife. She tells you that this morning he has been vomiting large amounts of fresh red blood and further questioning reveals an extensive alcohol history. You examine him and notice he is pale and peripherally shut down with a tachycardia of 120, hypotensive and seeming a bit confused.

a What are you worried about immediately? *1 mark*
b State four common causes of an upper GI bleed. *4 marks*
c Explain the pathophysiology behind the bleeding, according to the most likely diagnosis, given in his history. *3 marks*
d Give three aspects of your immediate management. *3 marks*
e Name three investigations you would request for this patient. *3 marks*

2 Jane is a 32-year-old female with ulcerative colitis which has previously been well controlled for the last 4 years. Unfortunately she now presents to you with a 5-day history of severe abdominal pain, persistent bloody diarrhoea which also contains mucus, and reports opening her bowels up to 15 times a day.

a Broadly identify five causes of diarrhoea, and give one example of each. *5 marks*
b Suggest three ways you will be able to assess the severity of her disease. *3 marks*
c Suggest three investigations you would request. *3 marks*
d How would you manage an acute attack of severe colitis? *2 marks*
e Identify two indications for considering surgical intervention. *2 marks*

Complete SAQs for Medical Finals By P. Stather et al, Published 2010 by
Blackwell Publishing, ISBN: 978-1-4501-8928-6.

3 Alexander is a 35-year-old male smoker who is known to suffer from Crohn's disease.

a Give three ways in which you can distinguish macroscopically between Crohn's disease and ulcerative colitis.   *3 marks*

b Identify four non-GI systems that may be affected by inflammatory bowel disease and give one example for each.   *4 marks*

c Suggest three treatment options for Alexander's condition.   *3 marks*

d Suggest two complications of Crohn's disease.   *2 marks*

4 Samantha, a 49-year-old lady, presents to you with a 2-month history of epigastric discomfort which is worse on lying down, bending and especially worse after her morning coffee. Her weekly trips to the Indian restaurant have also had to stop and she has had to change her diet.

a Give two red-flag symptoms you would enquire about.   *2 marks*

b Name four risk factors of GORD.   *4 marks*

c All investigations are reported as normal. Suggest three classes of drugs used for the medical management of GORD, give one example of each and explain briefly how each works.   *3 marks*

d Suggest two surgical techniques for managing GORD.   *2 marks*

e Give two complications of GORD.   *2 marks*

5 Balbir, a 69-year-old male who immigrated to the UK from the Middle East a few years ago, presents to you with progressive dysphagia which was initially only to food but now he is having difficulty with swallowing liquids. On examining him you notice tobacco stains, signs of malnourishment and his clothes are hung very loosely.

a What four questions would you like to ask him.   *4 marks*

b Give four risk factors for oesophageal carcinoma.   *2 marks*

c Give two ways in which you would investigate this patient.   *2 marks*

d Suggest four ways in which you would manage this patient.   *4 marks*

6 George, a 78-year-old retired miner, presents to you with several months' history of worsening epigastric pain, worse during eating, with partial relief after antacids.

   a What is the most likely diagnosis?   *1 mark*

   b Give three causes of this condition.   *3 marks*

   c Name two methods to identify *Helicobacter pylori*.   *2 marks*

   d What is the standard treatment of *H. pylori* infection?   *3 marks*

   e Give three complications of this patient's condition.   *3 marks*

7 Sumitra a 35-year old lady presents to you with long-standing diarrhoea, associated weight loss, general tiredness and abdominal pain which she has not seen anyone for. On examination she looks anaemic and a splint on her right hand is noticed where she sustained a fracture after a recent fall.

a   What is the diagnosis and aetiology?   2 marks

   b Give one pathological change you would find in this condition.   *1 mark*

   c Name four other causes of malabsorption in the small intestine.   *2 marks*

   d Give three investigations you would request in this patient.   *3 marks*

   e What dietary advice would you give the patient and what further investigation would you request to confirm the diagnosis?   *2 marks*

   f Name one long-term complication of this condition.   *1 mark*

8 Shania, a 38-year-old woman, presents to A & E with nausea, vomiting and malaise after taking 100 paracetamol tablets earlier that day.

   a Explain the pathophysiology of how paracetamol causes liver damage.   *2 marks*

   b What two blood tests would request in this patient?   *2 marks*

   c Give four ways in which you would manage this patient further.   *4 marks*

   d Name two complications of hepatic failure.   *2 marks*

   e Name a simple bedside test to assess encephalopathy.   *1 mark*

9 James, a 10-year-old boy who recently moved to the UK with his parents from Zambia, presents to you with a 14-day history of nausea, vomiting, diarrhoea and abdominal pain with a mild fever. On examination he is jaundiced and has hepatomegaly. After extensive investigation you make a diagnosis of hepatitis A.

a What is the pathology in hepatitis? *1 mark*

b Name two risk factors associated with
hepatitis A. *2 marks*

c Give three causes of acute and three causes of
chronic hepatitis. *6 marks*

d Which groups of people are at risk of
contracting hepatitis B infections *(2 marks)* and
what can be done for these groups *(1 marks)* *3 marks*

10 Peter, a 41-year-old male with long-term addiction to alcohol,
presents to you with abdominal distension, shortness of breath,
considerable weight gain and confusion. He is very well known
to the gastroenterology team and has long-standing liver
cirrhosis.

a Name eight further signs of liver disease. *4 marks*

b Suggest why ascites occurs in patients with
liver disease. *2 marks*

c What is the management of ascites and name
a complication. *1 mark*

d Differentiate between exudates and transudates. *2 marks*

e Given his alcohol history, what three medications
would you prescribe? *3 marks*

11 Frederick, a 45-year-old male, presents to you with a long-
standing history of loss of libido and joint pains. On examination he has bronze skin pigmentation and hepatomegaly.
Several investigations show high blood glucose, high serum
iron and ferritin levels, and deranged LFTs.

a Name three tests included in a liver function test. *3 marks*

b What is the likely diagnosis? *1 mark*

c Explain the pathology of the disease. *2 marks*

d Name two other organs that are affected. *2 marks*

e How is this disease managed? *2 marks*

12 Ingrid, a 17-year-old female student from Norway, presents to
you with signs of liver cirrhosis, a mild tremor and speech problems. On slit lamp examination, Kayser-Fleisher rings are seen.

a What is the likely diagnosis? *1 mark*

b Name three other clinical features of the disease. *3 marks*

c Explain the pathology of the disease. *3 marks*

d Name three investigations you would request. *3 marks*

e How would you treat the condition? *1 mark*

Gastroenterology

ANSWERS

1 a Hypovolaemic shock *(1 mark)*   ☐ /1
 b *(1 mark for each correct answer, maximum 4 marks)*   ☐ /4
   Oesophageal varices *(1 mark)*
   Gastritis *(1 mark)*
   Duodenal/gastric ulcer *(1 mark)*
   Mallory-Weiss tear *(1 mark)*
   Oesophagitis *(1 mark)*
   Malignancy *(1 mark)*
   Vascular malformation *(1 mark)*
   Duodentitis *(1 mark)*
 c Alcohol damages the liver causing cirrhosis *(1 mark)*   ☐ /3
   which disrupts the liver architecture and effectively
   acts as a tourniquet, reducing blood flow into
   the liver, which causes a build-up in pressure and
   portal hypertension *(1 mark)*. Some sites are more
   prone to the bleeding, due to superficial vessels in
   the gastro-oesophageal junction and rectum *(1 mark)*.
 d *(1 mark for each correct answer, maximum 3 marks)*   ☐ /3
   ABC *(1 mark)*
   IV access *(1 mark)*
   Fluid resuscitation and catheterise *(1 mark)*
   IV PPI in high-risk patients *(1 mark)*
   Senior support, surgeons, gastro team *(1 mark)*
   Sengstaken-Blakemore tube *(1 mark)*
 e Bloods (FBC, U+E, LFT, glucose, clotting screen,   ☐ /3
   group and X-match) *(1 mark)*
   Portable CXR *(1 mark)*
   Urgent OGD *(1 mark)*

Summary

Patients present with haemetemesis and may be haemodynami-
cally unstable. Initial management is to stabilise the patient prior
to endoscopic investigation. An upper GI bleed is a very common

presenting complaint, with the main three causes being peptic ulcer, oesophagitis and varices. Most bleeds stop spontaneously but require fluid resusucitation and possibly blood transfusions, with some requiring urgent surgery in order to stop the bleeding.

2 a Inflammatory bowel disease (Crohn's disease and
    ulcerative colitis) *(1 mark for category and example)*   `/5`
    Infective bacterial (*Staphylococcus, Campylobacter,*
    Salmonella, E coli) *(1 mark for category and example)*
    Infective viral (Rotavirus, CMV, Norwalk virus,
    HSV) *(1 mark for category and example)*
    Malignancy (colon cancer) *(1 mark for category*
    and example)
    Malabsorption (Coeliac disease, lactose intolerance,
    pernicious anaemia, short bowel syndrome)
    (1 mark for category and example)
    Parasites (Giardia lamblia, Entamoeba histolytics,
    Cryptosporidium) *(1 mark for category and example)*
    Medication (Antibiotics, Antacids) *(1 mark for*
    category and example)

b *(1 mark for each correct answer, maximum 3 marks)*   `/3`
    Stool frequency >6 per day *(1 mark)*
    Bloody diarrhoea *(1 mark)*
    Fever *(1 mark)*
    Tachycardia *(1 mark)*
    High ESR/CRP *(1 mark)*
    Anaemia *(1 mark)*
    Low albumin *(1 mark)*

c *(1 mark for each correct answer, maximum 3 marks)*   `/3`
    Blood tests (FBC, U+E, CRP, LFT, ESR, pANCA)
    (1 mark)
    Stool cultures *(1 mark)*
    AXR and erect CXR *(1 mark)*
    Abdominal CT/USS *(1 mark)*
    Sigmoidoscopy/colonoscopy *(1 mark)*

d *(1 mark for each correct answer, maximum 2 marks)*   `/2`
    Fluid and electrolyte support *(1 mark)*
    5-ASA compounds *(1 mark)*
    Steroids *(1 mark)*
    Ciclosporin *(1 mark)*
    LMWH *(1 mark)*
    Enemas *(1 mark)*

e *(1 mark for each correct answer, maximum 2 marks)* /2

Failure of medical treatment *(1 mark)*
Toxic dilatation *(1 mark)*
Haemorrhage *(1 mark)*
Perforation *(1 mark)*
Stricture *(1 mark)*
Obstruction *(1 mark)*

Summary

Ulcerative colitis is characterised by mucosal inflammation, which is not through the bowel wall. Presenting features are diarrhoea with blood and mucus and weight loss. The pathogenesis of this condition is unclear but a proposed theory suggests the role of environmental triggers in certain individuals who are genetically predisposed. 5-ASA compounds have a principal role in ulcerative colitis to maintain remission. Severe colitis is important to identify and manage quickly, with some complications requiring immediate surgical intervention, such as toxic megacolon.

3 a *(½ mark for each correct answer, maximum 3 marks)* /3

Crohn's disease: Affects anywhere from mouth to anus *(1 mark)*. Presence of skip lesions *(1 mark)*. Deep ulcers have a cobblestone appearance and penetrate transmurally *(1 mark)*.
Ulcerative colitis: Affects only colon *(1 mark)*. Extends proximally from rectum *(1 mark)*. Mucosal inflammation *(1 mark)*.

b *(1 mark for each correct answer, maximum 4 marks)* /4

Eyes: uveitis, episcleritis, conjunctivitis *(1 mark)*
Joints: small joint arthritis, ankylosing spondylitis, sacro-ileitis *(1 mark)*
Liver: cirrhosis, primary sclerosing cholangitis, chronic hepatitis, fatty change *(1 mark)*
Renal: calculi *(1 mark)*
Haematological: venous thrombosis, vasculitis *(1 mark)*

c *(1 mark for each correct answer, maximum 3 marks)* /3

Stop smoking *(1 mark)*
5-ASA compounds *(1 mark)*
Corticosteroids *(1 mark)*

Methotrexate *(1 mark)*
Cyclosporin *(1 mark)*
Azathioprine *(1 mark)*
Anti-TNF alpha *(1 mark)*
d *(1 mark for each correct answer, maximum 2 marks)* /2
Fissures *(1 mark)*
Fistulae *(1 mark)*
Haemorrhoids *(1 mark)*
Skin tags *(1 mark)*
Abscess *(1 mark)*
Strictures *(1 mark)*
Obstruction *(1 mark)*
Adhesions *(1 mark)*

Summary

Presenting features are similar to UC with abdominal pain, diarrhoea with blood and weight loss. Crohn's disease can affect any part of the gut from mouth to anus, with characteristically inflamed transmural patches. The diagnosis depends on finding graunulomatous asymmetric patches of inflammation. Crohn's disease patients tend to present with diarrhoea, weight loss and abdominal pain.

4 a *(1 mark for each correct answer, maximum 2 marks)* /2
Weight loss *(1 mark)*
Vomiting *(1 mark)*
Dysphagia *(1 mark)*
Symptoms of anaemia *(1 mark)*
Melaena *(1 mark)*

b *(1 mark for each correct answer, maximum 4 marks)* /4
Smoking *(1 mark)*
Alcohol *(1 mark)*
Spicy foods *(1 mark)*
Pregnancy *(1 mark)*
Obesity *(1 mark)*
Stress *(1 mark)*
Family history *(1 mark)*
Hiatus hernia *(1 mark)*

c *(1 mark for each correct answer, maximum 3 marks)* /3
Alginate agents, e.g. Gaviscon. This is an alkali which neutralises the acid. *(1 mark)*

H2RA, e.g. Ranitidine. Works by blocking the
secretion of acid. *(1 mark)*

PPI, e.g. omeprazole, inhibits the proton pump
responsible for secretion. *(1 mark)*

Prokinetic agents, e.g. metoclopramide, increase
frequency of gastric emptying. *(1 mark)*

d *(1 mark for each correct answer, maximum 2 marks)* /2

Endoscopy: Gastroplasty *(1 mark)*, endoscopic
injections *(1 mark)*

Surgery: Nissen's fundoplication *(1 mark)*

e *(1 mark for each correct answer, maximum 2 marks)* /2

Oesophageal stricture *(1 mark)*

Barrett's oesophagus *(1 mark)*

Oesophageal cancer *(1 mark)*

Chronic pain *(1 mark)*

Summary

Patients typically present with epigastric pain after eating spicy food and on lying down or stooping over. The pain of GORD occurs due to the reflux of gastric contents into the oesophagus causing irritation. Physiologically there is reduced tone in the lower oesophageal sphincter, permitting reflux back into the oesophagus, such as in hiatus hernia. If this continues it may lead to Barrett's Oesophagus, where there is an epithelial change from the normal squamous cells change to columnar epithelium.

5 a *(1 mark for each correct answer, maximum 4 marks)* /4

Enquire about the dysphagia. *(1 mark)*

Amount of weight loss? *(1 mark)*

Chest pain? *(1 mark)*

Shortness of breath? *(1 mark)*

Smoking and alcohol history? *(1 mark)*

Dietary history? *(1 mark)*

Family history of malignancy? *(1 mark)*

Past medical history? *(1 mark)*

Change in bowel habit? *(1 mark)*

b *(1 mark for each correct answer, maximum 4 marks)* /2

Alcohol *(1 mark)*

Smoking *(1 mark)*

Dietary (pickled vegetables) *(1 mark)*

GORD *(1 mark)*

Achalasia *(1 mark)*

Barrett's oesophagus *(1 mark)*

c *(1 mark for each correct answer, maximum 2 marks)*   /2
  Routine bloods *(1 mark)*
  Barium swallow/OGD + biopsy *(1 mark)*
  Staging CT/Staging MRI/PET scan *(1 mark)*
d *(1 mark for each correct answer, maximum 4 marks)*   /4
  Symptomatic treatment *(1 mark)*
  Dilatation of the stricture and insertion of a stent to
    keep the oesophagus open *(1 mark)*
  Laser to photocoagulate the tumour *(1 mark)*
  Alcohol injections into the tumour to cause local
    necrosis *(1 mark)*
  Assess nutrition: dietician review – may need
    NG tube or PEG *(1 mark)*
  Further imaging to stage (USS and CT) *(1 mark)*
  Surgery if tumour not infiltrated wall *(1 mark)*
  Neoadjuvant chemotherapy *(1 mark)*

Summary

Oesophageal cancer is more common in old age as nearly two-thirds of cases are diagnosed in patients over 65 years old. Patients may present with dysphagia, and the feeling of fullness in the throat. The disease is often extensively spread at time of diagnosis and carries a poor prognosis. The two major types of oesophageal cancer are squamous and adenocarcinoma. The primary symptom of oesophageal carcinoma is dysphagia and warrants urgent referral for endoscopy.

6 a Gastric ulcer disease *(1 mark)*   /1
  b *(1 mark for each correct answer, maximum 3 marks)*   /3
    H. pylori *(1 mark)*
    NSAIDs *(1 mark)*
    Alcohol *(1 mark)*
    Smoking *(1 mark)*
    Spicy food *(1 mark)*
    Stress *(1 mark)*
    Hyperparathyroidism *(1 mark)*
    Zollinger-Ellison syndrome *(1 mark)*
  c *(1 mark for each correct answer, maximum 2 marks)*   /2
    Urea breath test *(1 mark)*
    Endoscopy and histology *(1 mark)*
    Serological tests to detect IgG antibodies *(1 mark)*

H. pylori stool antigen *(1 mark)*
d A PPI *(1 mark)* and 2 antibiotics such as /3
clarithromycin *(1 mark)* + metronidazole/
amoxicillin *(1 mark)*
e *(1 mark for each correct answer, maximum 3 marks)* /3
Perforation *(1 mark)*
Gastric cancer *(1 mark)*
Haemorrhage *(1 mark)*
Anaemia *(1 mark)*
Chronic pain *(1 mark)*
Gastric outlet obstruction *(1 mark)*

Summary

Gastric ulcers present with epigastric pain which is worse on eating, whereas duodenal ulcers are relieved by eating. They are often caused by *Helicobacter pylori*, which is able to infect various areas of the stomach. It is able to survive in the stomach by producing urease, helping to form ammonia and carbon dioxide, which is then able to neutralise the gastric acid. It is thought that it is transmitted orally by contamination of food and water supplies, with most people acquiring the infection in early childhood. This is an important risk factor for the development of peptic ulcer disease and gastric cancer.

7 a Coeliac disease *(1 mark)* – an abnormal immune /2
response to alpha-gliadin within gluten (wheat)
products, causing abnormal jejunal mucosa
(gluten-sensitive enteropathy) *(1 mark)*. She may
have secondary osteoporosis due to this.
b *(maximum 1 mark)* /1
Subtotal villus atrophy *(1 mark)*
Chronic inflammatory cell infiltrate *(1 mark)*
Increased intraepithelial cell lymphocytes
(1 mark)
c *(½ mark for each correct answer, maximum 2 marks)* /2
Crohn's disease *(1 mark)*
Lactose intolerance *(1 mark)*
Intestinal resection *(1 mark)*
Small bowel bacterial overgrowth *(1 mark)*
Tropical sprue *(1 mark)*
Whipples disease *(1 mark)*

Parasitic infection *(1 mark)*
d *(1 mark for each correct answer, maximum 3 marks)*   /3
Jejunal mucosal biopsy *(1 mark)*
HLA typing *(1 mark)*
Biochemistry *(1 mark)*
Serum antibodies *(1 mark)*
Blood count *(1 mark)*
Small bowel follow-through *(1 mark)*
Bone densitometry *(1 mark)*
e Gluten-free diet *(1 mark)*   /2
Repeat biopsy after elimination of gluten
    containing foods would show improvement
    (1 mark)
f *(maximum 1 mark)*   /1
Intestinal lymphoma *(1 mark)*
Small bowel and oesophageal carcinoma *(1 mark)*
Anaemia *(1 mark)*
Osteoporosis *(1 mark)*

Summary

Coeliac disease is a common but underdiagnosed chronic inflammatory disease affecting the intestine which is genetically determined and induced by the substance gluten. Patients present with diarrhoea, weight loss, and steatorrhoea. It is associated with osteoporosis and malignancy. Patients need to be started on gluten-free diets and require referral to the dietician to promote health and correct other mineral deficiencies.

8 a *(1 mark for each correct answer, maximum 2 marks)*   /2
Paracetamol is converted to a toxic metabolite
    N-acetyl-p-benzoquinoneimine. *(1 mark)*
This is inactivated by glutathione. *(1 mark)*
In an overdose glutathione is depleted and the toxic
    metabolite accumulates causing necrosis of the
    hepatocytes. *(1 mark)*
b Clotting and LFT – liver function *(1 mark)*   /2
U&E – kidney function *(1 mark)*
c *(1 mark for each correct answer, maximum*   /4
    4 marks)
ABG *(1 mark)*
Activated charcoal if presents within 1 hr
    of ingestion *(1 mark)*

N-acetylcysteine according to protocol *(1 mark)*
Renal unit if develops ARF *(1 mark)*
Liver transplant unit if required *(1 mark)*
Refer to psychiatry *(1 mark)*

d *(1 mark for each correct answer, maximum 2 marks)* 〔 /2 〕
Cerebral oedema *(1 mark)*
Hypoglycaemia *(1 mark)*
Bleeding *(1 mark)*
Encephalopathy *(1 mark)*
Bacterial/fungal infections *(1 mark)*
Hypotension *(1 mark)*
Renal failure (hepatorenal syndrome) *(1 mark)*

e *(maximum 1 mark)* 〔 /1 〕
Draw a 5-pointed star *(1 mark)*
Draw concentric circles *(1 mark)*
Hepatic flap *(1 mark)*

Summary

Paracetamol overdose is the most common form of poisoning in the United Kingdom, either accidental or intentional. After it is ingested patients are often asymptomatic for the first 24 hours and liver damage is not usually detected until after 18–20 hours post ingestion. It causes deranged LFT's and clotting, which peaks at 72–96 hours post ingestion. Renal failure can also occur. N-Acetylcysteine is a very effective and protective agent if given within 8–10 hours of ingestion which works by replenishing the glutathione stores. Methionine can also be used to prevent hepatotoxicity in paracetamol overdose if used early, and there is currently debate over whether to include this in paracetamol preparations.

9 a *(maximum 1 mark)* 〔 /1 〕
Hepatocyte necrosis *(1 mark)*
Infiltration of inflamed cells into surrounding
area *(1 mark)*

b *(1 mark for each correct answer, maximum 2 marks)* 〔 /2 〕
Developing country *(1 mark)*
Contaminated water supply *(1 mark)*
Shellfish *(1 mark)*
Poor sanitation *(1 mark)*

c Acute – viruses *(1 mark)*, alcohol *(1 mark)*, drugs 〔 /6 〕
(1 mark), metabolic *(1 mark)*, *Toxoplasma (1 mark)*
(maximum 3 marks)

Chronic – viruses *(1 mark)*, autoimmune disease
(1 mark), alcohol *(1 mark)*, drugs *(1 mark)*
(maximum 3 marks)

d Healthcare workers *(1 mark)*, sex workers *(1 mark)*,   ☐ /3
IV drug users *(1 mark) (maximum 2 marks)*
Course of immunisations and regular boosters *(1 mark)*

Summary

The most common type of viral hepatitis is hepatitis A and tends to
affect children and young adults. It occurs worldwide and is spread
via the faecal to oral route in over crowded areas that have poor
access to sanitation and where food and water supplies are contaminated. It is a notifiable disease in the UK.

Hepatitis B is spread via the IV route and sexual contact as the
virus is present in semen and saliva. The most common transmission is vertically from mother to child during birth. The best form
of prevention is to avoid the risk factors and high-risk individuals,
such as hospital workers and sex workers, should be immunised.

10 a *(½ mark for each correct answer, maximum 4 marks)*   ☐ /4
Jaundice *(½ mark)*
Spider naevi *(½ mark)*
Gynaecomastia *(½ mark)*
Fetor hepaticus *(½ mark)*
Palmar erythema *(½ mark)*
Scratch marks *(½ mark)*
Parotitis *(½ mark)*
Purpura *(½ mark)*
Hepatic flap *(½ mark)*
Coma *(½ mark)*
Ascites *(½ mark)*
Visible veins *(½ mark)*

b *(1 mark for each correct answer, maximum 2 marks)*   ☐ /2
Activated renin angiotensin aldosterone
system *(1 mark)*
Salt and water retention *(1 mark)*
Hypoalbuminaemia *(1 mark)*
Increased toxic metabolites as liver has decreased
function causing vasodilatation *(1 mark)*

c Ascitic tap/drain *(½ mark)*   ☐ /1
Spontaneous bacterial peritonitis *(½ mark)*

d Transudate (low protein content): cirrhosis, /2
constrictive pericarditis, cardiac failure, renal
failure *(1 mark)*
Exudate (high protein content): malignancy,
infection, pancreatitis, Budd-Chiari syndrome,
myxoedema, lymphatic obstruction *(1 mark)*

e High-strength vitamin B *(1 mark)* /3
Chlordiazepoxide-reducing regime *(1 mark)*
Thiamine *(1 mark)*

Summary
Ascites occurs in over half of cirrhotic patients over a 10-year period and is associated with an increased mortality. Other major causes of ascites include malignancy and heart failure. The commonest site for an ascitic tap is 15 cm lateral to the umbilicus and the sample obtained should be screened for the possible development of spontaneous bacterial peritonitis which can occur in 15% of liver cirrhosis patients. It is diagnostic if neutrophil count is >250 cells/mm^3.

11 a *(1 mark for each correct answer, maximum 3 marks)* /3
Bilirubin *(1 mark)*
ALT *(1 mark)*
Alkaline phosphatase *(1 mark)*
GGT *(1 mark)*
AST *(1 mark)*
Albumin *(1 mark)*
Total protein *(1 mark)*

b Hereditary haemochromatosis *(1 mark)* /1

c *(1 mark for each correct answer, maximum 2 marks)* /2
Autosomal recessive *(1 mark)*
HFE gene mutation *(1 mark)*
Excessive iron absorption from small bowel *(1 mark)*
Excess iron deposition in various organs *(1 mark)*

d *(1 mark for each correct answer, maximum 2 marks)* /2
Heart *(1 mark)*
Pancreas *(1 mark)*
Pituitary gland *(1 mark)*

e Venesection *(1 mark)* /2
Desferoximine *(1 mark)*

Summary

Hereditary haemochromatosis is a genetic condition causing excess absorption and deposition of iron into tissues. These patients have very high levels of total body iron of around 30 g, with higher levels occurring in the pancreas and liver. They may have a slate-grey appearance. Complications of this disease include cirrhosis, hepatocellular carcinoma and diabetes.

12 a Wilson's disease *(1 mark)* `/1`
  b *(1 mark for each correct answer, maximum 3 marks)* `/3`
   Liver disease *(1 mark)*
   Tremor *(1 mark)*
   Speech problems *(1 mark)*
   Dementia *(1 mark)*
   Haemolytic anaemia *(1 mark)*
   Renal tubular defects *(1 mark)*
  c Autosomal recessive *(1 mark)* `/3`
   Failure of biliary copper excretion *(1 mark)*
   Copper is deposited in liver, basal ganglia
     and cornea *(1 mark)*
  d Serum copper and caeruloplasmin *(1 mark)* `/3`
   Urinary copper (24 hr) *(1 mark)*
   Liver biopsy *(1 mark)*
  e *(maximum 1 mark)* `/1`
   Penicillamine – chelates copper to enhance its
     excretion *(1 mark)*
   Liver transplant *(1 mark)*
   Relative screening *(1 mark)*

Summary

Patients tend to present with neurological and hepatic problems in Wilson's disease, where there is an error in the copper metabolism pathway resulting in the deposition of copper in various organs including the liver, brain and cornea. The disease occurs worldwide but particularly in countries where consanguinity is prevalent. It is important that all young patients with liver disease are screened as these patients can be treated and their outlook improved.

4 Neurology

QUESTIONS

1 A 72-year-old lady comes to your surgery with her daughter. She tells you that 2 days ago while out shopping she felt her left leg go weak and had to sit down quickly. A shop assistant came over to her and asked if she was alright, but the patient was unable to get her words out and her speech was slurred. She reports having felt dizzy but that her symptoms resolved within a couple of hours. You suspect she might have suffered a TIA.

a List two differential diagnoses.	*2 marks*
b What is the definition of a TIA?	*1 mark*
c Name three risk factors for a TIA.	*3 marks*
d Name three investigations you would like to request.	*3 marks*
e Your investigations show that her right carotid artery is 70% stenosed. You refer her to the vascular surgeon. What three other aspects of management would you initiate?	*3 marks*
f Name two other conditions that are associated with vascular disease above the level of the chest.	*2 marks*

2 A 22-year-old girl comes to see you saying that she has been experiencing throbbing headaches. On further questioning she says that the pain is usually on one side of her head and that she usually vomits at least once. The headaches last for about a day and she has had to have time off work.

a What is the most likely diagnosis?	*1 mark*
b Give three other questions you would ask to confirm your diagnosis.	*3 marks*

Complete SAQs for Medical Finals By P. Stather et al, Published 2010 by Blackwell Publishing, ISBN: 978-1-4501-8928-6.

c If she had tension headaches how would she
  describe the pain?   *1 mark*

d What are the two most serious differential
  diagnoses you must exclude before you can
  diagnose your answer to part a)?   *2 marks*

e Suggest two examinations you would do to try
  to exclude these.   *2 marks*

f The diagnosis in this case is a clinical one. You
  explain this to the patient. How would you treat
  her in the acute phase   *2 marks*
  and long term?   *2 marks*

3 A 75-year-old lady comes to your general medical outpatient
clinic with problems with her mobility. She says that she has
difficulty standing up from a chair and has suffered two falls
recently. She has also noticed a slight tremor in her hands.

a What three other questions would you want to ask?   *3 marks*

b You suspect Parkinson's disease. What is the triad
  of clinical features experienced in this condition?   *1 mark*

c What other four clinical features might you find
  in your patient?   *4 marks*

d Briefly outline the pathology of Parkinson's disease.   *2 marks*

e Give four ways you could manage a patient
  with newly diagnosed Parkinson's disease.   *4 marks*

4 An 84-year-old lady is brought into A & E by ambulance after suddenly collapsing at her neighbour's house. She is conscious but not
responsive to questioning. On examination she exhibits increased
tone and immobility of her left arm and leg, and is hyper-reflexive
there too. You feel it is likely that she has had a stroke.

a What are the two main types of stroke in terms
  of pathophysiology?   *1 mark*

b Given the history above, what blood supply is
  most likely to be implicated?   *1 mark*

c Give four ways in which you would initially
  manage this patient.   *4 marks*

d Investigations reveal that the patient has suffered
  a cerebral infarct. Her GCS is stable at 15/15.
  What three things would you do now with regard
  to further management?   *3 marks*

e Apart from doctors and nurses, name four
  members of the multidisciplinary team who
  can help with the care of stroke patients.   *2 marks*

f Your patient has been in hospital now for 2 months whilst her social care arrangements are finalised. Suggest three possible complications from her stroke. *3 marks*

5 A 26-year-old man comes to A & E after suffering a seizure at home witnessed by his girlfriend. She reported that he suddenly went rigid, his eyes rolled back and then he started to shake. She is not aware of him ever having suffered a seizure before or any medical history. The patient is drowsy but responsive and appears to be a bit confused.

   a What is the name given to this type of seizure? *1 mark*
   b The patient is not able to give a history and his girlfriend cannot tell you any more. What three things would you do next? *3 marks*
   c Name four possible causes of a seizure in this patient. *4 marks*
   d Name two other common side-effects of carbamazepine. *2 marks*
   e Apart from treating seizures name one other condition carbamazepine can be used to treat. *1 mark*
   f The patient's girlfriend takes you to one side and asks you what is the matter with him. What do you tell her? *1 mark*
   g Name two implications of being diagnosed with epilepsy apart from the side-effects of anti-epileptics. *2 marks*

6 A 30-year-old woman comes to see you saying that she woke up this morning with blurred vision. She also had excruciating pain around her left eye, made worse when she moves her eye. Ten months previously she had come to see you with numbness and parasthesia in her left leg but this resolved completely within 3 days. You suspect multiple sclerosis.

   a Give two other differential diagnoses. *2 marks*
   b Give three aspects of your management of this patient. *3 marks*
   c To complete your history what three other symptoms would you enquire about? *3 marks*
   d A diagnosis of MS is made. What tracts in the brain are responsible for sensory symptoms in her left leg? *2 marks*
   e Some patients present with internuclear opthalmoplegia. What is this? *1 mark*
   f Briefly outline the pathophysiology of MS. *2 marks*

7 A 50-year-old woman is admitted to A & E with an intense headache which started suddenly about half an hour ago. She has vomited twice and was unable to stand up as the pain is so severe. Her husband said that she has had a few headaches over the past weeks that have responded to simple analgesia and rest. You suspect a subarachnoid haemorrhage.

   a What two other differential diagnoses would you be considering from this history?   *2 marks*

   b You arrange a CT scan which shows SAH. If this had been negative for SAH but you still suspected this, what other investigation would you order that might confirm it?   *1 mark*

   c Name the three layers of the meninges, outermost first.   *3 marks*

   d Is a bleed into the subarachnoid space a venous or arterial bleed?   *1 mark*

   e Name two causes of SAH.   *2 marks*

   f What is the definitive treatment for SAH?   *1 mark*

   g Name two complications of SAH.   *2 marks*

8 A 73-year-old gentleman presents with a headache that has come on suddenly. He does not report any head injury. He says he is tired and appears drowsy. He is not oriented to time or place. He was previously fit, well and independent.

   a What three things would you do initially for this patient?   *3 marks*

   b From this history, apart from a subdural haematoma two other serious conditions you would want to exclude.   *2 marks*

   c Is a subdural bleed venous or arterial in origin?   *1 mark*

   d Between which layers of the meninges does the haematoma develop?   *1 mark*

   e Name three risk factors for developing a subdural bleed.   *3 marks*

   f Radiological imaging shows that the patient has a subdural bleed. What would you do now?   *1 mark*

   g What is the definitive treatment?   *1 mark*

9 A 35-year-old man comes to see you with numbness and parasthesiae in his fingers and toes. It is sometimes accompanied by pain. He has had diabetes since childhood. He gets these symptoms on most days.

   a Describe the distribution of his symptoms.   *1 mark*

b On examination you notice some wasting of the
distal muscle groups. Which three other features
would you expect to find on examination? *3 marks*

c What is your most likely diagnosis? *1 mark*

d Name four other causes of this condition. *4 marks*

e Give three ways in which you would manage this
patient. *3 marks*

10 A 19-year-old university student comes to see you with a worsening severe headache which she has had for about 10 hours. She has had flu-like symptoms for about the same length of time. She has recently developed stiffness in her neck and photophobia. Her housemates bring her in to see you as they think she might have meningitis.

a Name two common organisms that can cause
meningitis in this age group of patients. *2 marks*

b Name two investigations apart from blood tests
you would request, in what order, and why? *2 marks*

c Describe three differences seen on analysis of the
CSF between viral and bacterial meningitis. *3 marks*

d Apart from investigations give three points on
how you would manage this patient. *3 marks*

e Name three common, long-term complications
of bacterial meningitis. *3 marks*

11 A 34-year-old woman comes into A & E having collapsed suddenly at home. She has been feeling increasingly weak and tired for the past few months; this is worse at the end of the day. She also reports difficulty with swallowing food and has felt that she is mildly short of breath at rest on occasion despite being fit and active up to a few months ago.

a Name three non-neurological differential diagnoses. *3 marks*

b You notice that she exhibits myopathic facies.
Name three specific features of this. *3 marks*

c Your registrar suggests myasthenia gravis. What two
other observations might you make from inspection
that would be consistent with this diagnosis? *2 marks*

d Name two tests you could request to confirm this
diagnosis and describe it. *2 marks*

e Give three ways in which you would manage
this patient once myasthenia gravis has been
diagnosed? *3 marks*

Neurology

ANSWERS

1 a *(1 mark for each correct answer, maximum 2 marks)* ☐ /2
  Hypoglycaemic episode *(1 mark)*
  Social anxiety *(1 mark)*
  Postural hypotension *(1 mark)*
b A sudden loss of focal CNS function that resolves ☐ /1
  within 24 hours *(1 mark)*
c *(1 mark for each correct answer, maximum 3 marks)* ☐ /3
  Smoking *(1 mark)*
  Diabetes *(1 mark)*
  Hypertension *(1 mark)*
  Age *(1 mark)*
  Previous TIA *(1 mark)*
  Hyperlipidaemia *(1 mark)*
  Ischaemic heart disease *(1 mark)*
  Heart valve abnormalities *(1 mark)*
  Coagulopathy *(1 mark)*
d *(1 mark for each correct answer, maximum 3 marks)* ☐ /3
  ECG – looking for AF or MI *(1 mark)*
  Carotid artery Doppler ultrasound *(1 mark)*
  FBC – looking for polycythaemia *(1 mark)*
  ESR – can be raised in endocarditis and vasculitis
    (1 mark)
  U&E *(1 mark)*
  CT/MRI brain *(1 mark)*
  Echocardiogram *(1 mark)*
  Fasting blood lipids and cholesterol *(1 mark)*
  Glucose *(1 mark)*
  Autoantibody profile *(1 mark)*
e *(1 mark for each correct answer, maximum 3 marks)* ☐ /3
  Start on statin and aspirin *(1 mark)*
  Advise her to lose weight if she is obese *(1 mark)*
  Stop smoking and drinking alcohol to excess *(1 mark)*
  Increase activity levels *(1 mark)*
  Optimise diabetic control if appropriate *(1 mark)*

f *(1 mark for each correct answer, maximum 2 marks)* ☐ /2
Stroke *(1 mark)*
Vascular dementia *(1 mark)*
Amaurosis fugax/retinal artery occlusion *(1 mark)*

Summary

The features in a TIA depend on which arterial territory is disrupted. If it lies within the carotid system then amaurosis fugax, aphasia, hemiparesis and hemianopic visual defects are more likely. If the event occurs in the vertebrobasilar system then ataxia, dysarthria, diplopia and vomiting can be experienced, as this system supplies the posterior aspect of the brain.

2 a Migraine *(1 mark)* ☐ /1
  b *(1 mark for each correct answer, maximum 3 marks)* ☐ /3
Any photophobia? *(1 mark)*
Visual problems accompanying the headache such
  as scotoma, unilateral blindness, flashing lights?
  (1 mark)
Any aphasia, tingling, numbness, weakness on one
  side of the body? *(1 mark)*
Any trigger factors? These can include foods
  (especially chocolate, cheese), post-stress and
  pre-menstruation *(1 mark)*
Recently started the OCP? *(1 mark)*
Any family history of migraines? *(1 mark)*
  c A pressure or tightness all around the head with no ☐ /1
  associated features *(1 mark)*
  d Meningitis *(1 mark)* ☐ /2
Brain tumour *(1 mark)*
  e *(1 mark for each correct answer, maximum 2 marks)* ☐ /2
Look for papilloedema *(1 mark)*
Examine the cranial nerves *(1 mark)*
Look for Kernig's sign and Brudzinski's sign
  (1 mark)
  f *(1 mark for each correct answer, maximum 2 marks for* ☐ /4
  acute phase and 2 marks for long-term treatment)
Treatment of an acute attack – simple analgesics and
  anti-emetics *(1 mark)*
Stop the combined oral contraceptive pill and suggest
  alternative contraception *(1 mark)*

Triptans – e.g. Sumatriptan. These are 5-HT1 agonists
and constrict the cranial arteries *(1 mark)*
Prophylaxis – indicated when patient experiencing
more than 2 attacks a month, which do not
respond to the above *(1 mark)*
Beta-blockers *(1 mark)*
Serotonin antagonists – Pizotifen *(1 mark)*
Amytriptyline *(1 mark)*
Avoidance of triggers *(1 mark)*

Summary

The pathogenesis of migraines has yet to be discovered, although
it is thought to be caused by vasodilatation of the extracerebral
vessels in the scalp and dura. At least 10% of the population
are thought to experience at least one migraine in their lifetime.
Typical age of onset is in the teenage years or early 20's. Women
are affected more than men.

3 a *(1 mark for each correct answer, maximum 3 marks)*   /3
When were the difficulties first noticed? *(1 mark)*
Any difficulty turning around in bed? *(1 mark)*
Independent with all ADLs? *(1 mark)*
Any recent or past head injuries? *(1 mark)*
Currently on any psychotrophic medications? – these
can give rise to extrapyramidal signs *(1 mark)*
Any depression or memory problems? – depression
and dementia can occur in later stages *(1 mark)*
Any associated symptoms of constipation, dysphagia,
or dribbling of saliva? *(1 mark)*
b Bradykinesia, rigidity and tremor *(1 mark)*   /1
c *(1 mark for each correct answer, maximum 4 marks)*   /4
Mask-like facies – lack of facial expression *(1 mark)*
Lack of spontaneous movements *(1 mark)*
Greasy skin – due to autonomic dysfunction *(1 mark)*
Decreased blinking *(1 mark)*
Titubation – nodding head involuntarily *(1 mark)*
Dribbling of saliva *(1 mark)*
Festinating gait *(1 mark)*
Cogwheel rigidity *(1 mark)*
Micrographia *(1 mark)*
Increased tone *(1 mark)*
Stooped posture *(1 mark)*

d Dopaminergic neurones projecting from the `/2` substantia nigra of the midbrain to the basal ganglia are damaged *(1 mark)*. This leads to an imbalance in the EPS to favour cholinergic and other neurotransmitters. *(1 mark)*

e *(1 mark for each correct answer, maximum 4 marks)* `/4`
Medications: L-Dopa – most oral L-dopa is metabolised to dopamine before crossing the blood–brain barrier *(1 mark)*
Peripheral dopa decarboxylase inhibitor such as carbidopa to slow the metabolism of L-dopa – this has the benefit of reducing side-effects of L-dopa such as nausea and hypotension. One of the combinations is co-carbidopa *(1 mark)*
Other drugs include dopamine receptor agonists, anticholinergics and COMT inhibitors *(1 mark)*
SSRIs are the drug of choice for depression *(1 mark)*
Physiotherapy, to prevent falls, and involve other healthcare professionals such as occupational therapists and speech therapists *(1 mark)*
Neurosurgery – this is only used selectively and in younger patients *(1 mark)*
Information and support is provided by the Parkinson's Disease Society *(1 mark)*

Summary

L-Dopa becomes less effective over time, even with increasing doses. Motor fluctuations, either 'on-off phenomena' or abrupt wearing off of the drug, leaving the patient rigid and immobile, complicate treatment. Also dyskinesias (involuntary movements when dopamine levels are high) may occur. Co-careldopa is associated with confusion, delusions and hallucinations which may be so distressing that the patient ceases treatment.

4 a Haemorrhagic *(1 mark)* `/1`
Thromboembolic *(1 mark)*
 b The area that is supplied by the anterior `/1` cerebral artery *(1 mark)*
 c *(1 mark for each correct answer, maximum 4 marks)* `/4`

Reassure the patient, who will be very anxious even
though she might not be able to convey this to you
(1 mark)

Monitor GCS *(1 mark)*

CT/MRI brain – to distinguish between
thromboembolic, haemorrhagic, or neither *(1 mark)*

Bloods: glucose – looking for hypo- or hyperglycaemia,
U&E, FBC – looking for polycythaemia, INR – if
taking warfarin, ESR *(1 mark)*

ECG – AF or MI *(1 mark)*

NBM *(1 mark)*

d *(1 mark for each correct answer, maximum 3 marks)*　　　/3

Start aspirin, 300 mg daily *(1 mark)*

Consider giving thrombolysis. This improves outcome
if given within 3 hours of onset of symptoms of
acute stroke *(1 mark)*

Refer to a stroke unit *(1 mark)*

Monitor BP – do not treat any hypertension initially,
as a reduction in arterial pressure may cause
harmful decreases in local brain perfusion giving
rise to 'watershed infarcts' *(1 mark)*

Secondary prevention of further strokes: aspirin, statin,
smoking cessation, good glycaemic control if diabetic,
warfarin if in AF *(1 mark for each/maximum 1 mark)*

e *(½ mark for each correct answer, maximum 2 marks)*　　　/2

Physiotherapists *(½ mark)*

Occupational therapists *(½ mark)*

Speech and language therapists – not only for speech
therapy but they can also assess a patient's ability to
swallow which can be impaired after a stroke *(½ mark)*

Dietician *(½ mark)*

Social workers *(½ mark)*

Care assistants *(½ mark)*

Counsellors *(½ mark)*

f *(1 mark for each correct answer, maximum 3 marks)*　　　/3

Infection – pneumonia, UTI, septicaemia *(1 mark)*

Thromboembolism – PE, DVT *(1 mark)*

Hydration and nutritional difficulties *(1 mark)*

Seizures *(1 mark)*

Pressure sores *(1 mark)*

Spasticity with pain and/or contractures *(1 mark)*

Depression *(1 mark)*

Summary

About a quarter of patients die within the first 2 years of having a stroke. About a third of stroke patients will be permanently dependant on others for self-care and 10% will have a second stroke within 12 months. The prognosis for infarcts is better than for bleeds. Presenting symptoms depend greatly on the area and size of the infarction, ranging from a minor degree of weakness to coma. MRI is now the gold standard imaging modality, although this is not always practical due to its restricted availability. The difference between a TIA and a stroke is that symptoms must be completely resolved within 24 hours in a TIA. This can obviously make the diagnosis difficult early on.

5 a Tonic-clonic *(1 mark)* `/1`

  b *(1 mark for each correct answer, maximum 3 marks)* `/3`
   Ask for a full set of observations including capillary
     glucose *(1 mark)*
   Request patient's previous medical notes
     (1 mark)
   NBM *(1 mark)*
   Bloods – FBC, U&E, CRP, glucose, calcium and
     magnesium levels *(maximum 1 mark)*
   Monitor closely with a fit chart *(1 mark)*
   Obtain full history when he is awake *(1 mark)*
   Check for other injuries (secondary survey)
     (1 mark)
   CT head if appropriate *(1 mark)*

  c *(1 mark for each correct answer, maximum 4 marks)* `/4`
   Epilepsy – first episode or known epilepsy and not
     compliant with treatment *(1 mark)*
   Alcohol intoxication or withdrawal *(1 mark)*
   Infections – bacterial meningitis and encephalitis
     (1 mark)
   Head trauma *(1 mark)*
   Drugs – MAOIs, illicit *(1 mark)*
   Hypoxia *(1 mark)*
   Degenerative disease *(1 mark)*
   Sickle cell crisis *(1 mark)*
   Metabolic disturbance – hypocalcaemia,
     hypernatraemia, hypo/hypermagnesaemia
     (1 mark)
   Intracranial tumours *(1 mark)*

Toxins – carbon monoxide, iron, mercury *(1 mark)*
In his previous medical notes you read that the
patient has a history of epilepsy but has not
attended his last 2 appointments with his
neurologist. The patient is more alert now and
tells you that he was taking carbamazepine but
stopped taking it 2 months ago as it was causing
him to develop breasts and he was embarrassed.

d *(1 mark for each correct answer, maximum 2 marks)*   `/2`
Dizziness *(1 mark)*
Skin rash *(1 mark)*
Leucopenia *(1 mark)*
Nausea and vomiting *(1 mark)*
Ataxia *(1 mark)*
Visual disturbances *(1 mark)*
Inactivates the OCP *(1 mark)*
It is teratogenic *(1 mark)*

e *(1 mark for each correct answer, maximum 1 mark)*   `/1`
Prophylaxis of bipolar disorder *(1 mark)*
Trigeminal neuralgia *(1 mark)*

f Nothing as you must respect the patient's   `/1`
confidentiality *(1 mark)*

g *(1 mark for each correct answer, maximum 2 marks)*   `/2`
Driving is only permitted after 1 year being seizure
free – DVLA must be informed *(1 mark)*
Cannot drive heavy goods vehicles *(1 mark)*
Unable to work in the armed forces, as an aircraft
pilot, or as a train driver *(1 mark)*
Outdoor pursuits such as rock and tree climbing
should be restricted to situations where there is
adequate supervision *(1 mark)*
Have showers not baths in case of seizure *(1 mark)*

Summary

No cause is found for 75% of patients with epilepsy although
there is often a strong family history for developing it. Medications
should not be given after a single seizure, but a referral to a neurologist should be made.

There are several types of seizure, including tonic clonic, partial complex, partial simple, and absence seizures. An EEG is often
used to make the diagnosis, possibly with the need for 24-hour
studies.

6 a *(1 mark for each correct answer, maximum 2 marks)* `/2`
  TIA *(1 mark)*
  Migraine *(1 mark)*
  Brain tumour *(1 mark)*
 b *(1 mark for each correct answer, maximum 3 marks)* `/3`
  Admit patient to neurology ward or obtain
    neurology opinion *(1 mark)*
  MRI scan *(1 mark)*
  Visual evoked potentials – delayed-slow conduction
    on central white matter *(1 mark)*
  Analgesia *(1 mark)*
  A short course of corticosteroids *(1 mark)*
 c *(1 mark for each correct answer, maximum 3 marks)* `/3`
  Incontinence *(1 mark)*
  Difficulty walking *(1 mark)*
  Fatigue *(1 mark)*
  Paralysis *(1 mark)*
 d Spinothalamic tracts *(1 mark)* `/2`
  Posterior columns *(1 mark)*
 e Successful abduction on attempted lateral gaze but `/1`
  failure of adduction of the other eye causes
  double vision *(1 mark)*
 f *(1 mark for each correct answer, maximum 2 marks)* `/2`
  Demyelination of the white matter of the CNS
    (1 mark) that tends to favour the optic nerves,
    brainstem, periventricular areas and spinal cord
    (1 mark). Demyelination decreases conduction
    velocity and some of the signal dissipates
    causing information to be lost. *(1 mark)*

Summary

Favourable prognostic factors are, being female, less than 35 years at onset, having a single rather than multiple areas of CNS involvement and experiencing a complete recovery after an exacerbation. Less favourable prognostic factors are exhibiting brainstem symptoms such as tremor, nystagmus, and ataxia, as well as experiencing more frequent attacks. MS is seen with increasing frequency at areas of greater latitude.

7 a *(1 mark for each correct answer, maximum 2 marks)* `/2`
  Meningitis *(1 mark)*

Brain tumour *(1 mark)*
Migraine *(1 mark)*
b *(1 mark for each correct answer, maximum 1 mark)*   □ /1
Lumbar puncture – it must be performed at least
6 hours post symptom onset *(1 mark)*
Xanthochromia of the supernatant after
centrifugation of the CSF is diagnostic *(1 mark)*
c Dura mater *(1 mark)*   □ /3
Arachnoid mater *(1 mark)*
Pia mater *(1 mark)*
d Arterial *(1 mark)*   □ /1
e *(1 mark for each correct answer, maximum 2 marks)*   □ /2
Rupture of a berry aneurysm (70%) *(1 mark)*
Congenital AV malformations (10%) *(1 mark)*
Trauma *(1 mark)*
Vessels weakened by infection – septic emboli from
infective endocarditis *(1 mark)*
Coagulopathies *(1 mark)*
f Obliteration of the aneurysm by surgical clipping   □ /1
or insertion of a fine wire coil under radiological
guidance *(1 mark)*
g *(1 mark for each correct answer, maximum 2 marks)*   □ /2
Rebleeding *(1 mark)*
Hydrocephalus *(1 mark)*
Stroke *(1 mark)*
Death *(1 mark)*

Summary

Subarachnoid haemorrhage typically presents with a sudden headache which is often occipital, with neck stiffness, nausea, and focal neurology. About 50% of patients die suddenly or soon after the haemorrhage. A further 10–20% die from rebleeding in the early weeks in hospital. Outcome is variable in the survivors. Some have severe neurological deficits whereas others have only minor problems.

8 a *(1 mark for each correct answer, maximum 3 marks)*   □ /3
Full set of observations including BM *(1 mark)*
Full neurological examination including fundoscopy
(1 mark)
ABC *(1 mark)*
CT scan *(1 mark)*
NBM and cannulate *(1 mark)*

b *(1 mark for each correct answer, maximum 2 marks)* /2
Stroke *(1 mark)*
Intoxicated/drug overdose *(1 mark)*
Metabolic imbalance – hypoglycaemic *(1 mark)*
Septicaemia *(1 mark)*
Acute bleed into a brain tumour *(1 mark)*
c Venous *(1 mark)* /1
d Dura and arachnoid *(1 mark)* /1
e *(1 mark for each correct answer, maximum 3 marks)* /3
Increasing age – brain shrinkage occurs *(1 mark)*
Chronic alcoholism *(1 mark)*
Epilepsy *(1 mark)*
Long-term anticoagulation *(1 mark)*
Falls *(1 mark)*
f Refer to neurosurgery *(1 mark)* /1
g Surgical evacuation of the haematoma through /1
burr holes *(1 mark)*

Summary
A subdural haemorrhage can cause a rise in intracranial pressure. This can crush brain tissue, shift brain structures and cause the brain to herniate. Hence if a subdural haemorrhage is suspected a CT scan should be ordered to look for this or to rule out coning before a lumbar puncture is done as this can lead to further coning. Coning gives rise to brain ischaemia in the basal ganglia, leading to respiratory depression and death.

9 a Glove and stocking *(1 mark)* /1
b *(1 mark for each correct answer, maximum 3 marks)* /3
Reduced light touch and pin prick sensation limited
to his hands and feet *(1 mark)*
Absent or reduced ankle jerks *(1 mark)*
Loss of proprioception at level of the toes *(1 mark)*
Loss of vibration sense up to level of knees or iliac
crests *(1 mark)*
Pes cavus *(1 mark)*
Charcot joints *(1 mark)*
High-stepping gait – due to weakness of ankle
dorsiflexion *(1 mark)*
c Peripheral neuropathy secondary to diabetes /1
mellitus *(1 mark)*
d *(1 mark for each correct answer, maximum 4 marks)* /4

Vitamin B deficiency *(1 mark)*
Paraneoplastic *(1 mark)*
Alcohol abuse *(1 mark)*
Connective tissue disease/vasculitis such as SLE
   (1 mark)
Guillian Barre syndrome *(1 mark)*
Friedreich's ataxia *(1 mark)*
Hereditary motor-sensory neuropathy
   (Charcot-Marie-Tooth disease) *(1 mark)*
HIV *(1 mark)*
Drugs such as metronidazole and vincristine *(1 mark)*

e *(1 mark for each correct answer, maximum 3 marks)*   /3
Advise on how to optimise blood glucose control
   (1 mark)
Advise to wear sensible shoes or likely to get foot
   ulcers *(1 mark)*
Refer to podiatrist *(1 mark)*
Advise to avoid extremes of temperatures or likely
   to damage skin and deeper tissues *(1 mark)*
Bloods – FBC, ESR, Vit B12, U&E, HbA1c
   (maximum 1 mark)
Use atypical analgesics such as amitriptyline or
   gabapentin for pain rather than simple analgesics
   (1 mark)

Summary

Once diabetic neuropathy has set in it is irreversible. Patients should receive good foot care to prevent the development of foot ulcers, which are more likely to occur when the patient has reduced sensation and cannot detect pain.

At this stage it is important to prevent the condition worsening. Other causes that may be co-existing should be looked for. The above blood tests should rule out other common causes.

10 a *(1 mark for each correct answer, maximum 2 marks)*   /2
Neisseria meningitides (1 mark)
Streptococcus pneumoniae (1 mark)
Enteroviruses *(1 mark)*
Mycobacterium tuberculosis (1 mark)

b CT scan *(1 mark)* then lumbar puncture *(1 mark)*   /2
to rule out coning prior to the procedure.

c *(1 mark for each correct answer, maximum 3 marks)*   /3

Viral – pressure may be raised. Bacterial – pressure is often raised *(1 mark)*

Viral – appearance is clear. Bacterial – appearance is cloudy *(1 mark)*

Viral – glucose levels are normal. Bacterial – glucose levels are low *(1 mark)*

Viral – protein levels are low (<1.5 g/L). Bacterial – protein levels are high (>1.5 g/L) *(1 mark)*

Viral – predominant cells are polynuclear. Bacterial – predominant cells are polymorphs *(1 mark)*

Viral – no organisms seen in smear or culture. Bacterial – organisms may be seen in smear or culture *(1 mark)*

d *(1 mark for each correct answer, maximum 3 marks)* `/3`

Analgesia *(1 mark)*

Position the patient head up *(1 mark)*

IV benzylpenicillin if bacterial meningitis is suspected *(1 mark)*

Put patient in a darkened room in a quiet environment *(1 mark)*

e *(1 mark for each correct answer, maximum 3 marks)* `/3`

Hydrocephalus *(1 mark)*

Brain abscess *(1 mark)*

Epilepsy *(1 mark)*

Focal neurological deficits such as hearing impairment *(1 mark)*

Hemi and quadraparesis *(1 mark)*

Distal limb loss in septicaemia *(1 mark)*

Summary

Meningitis typically presents with headache, photophobia, neck stiffness, and a rash, and patients often have a positive Kernig's and Brudzinski's signs. It is recommended that all people under the age of 25 be vaccinated against meningitis C, which tends to occur in small outbreaks such as in schools. People who have been in close contact with someone who has been diagnosed with types A or C bacterial meningitis should be vaccinated against that particular type.

11 a *(1 mark for each correct answer, maximum 3 marks)* `/3`

aemia *(1 mark)*

Malignancy *(1 mark)*

Cardiac failure *(1 mark)*

Depression/anxiety *(1 mark)*

b *(1 mark for each correct answer, maximum 3 marks)* /3

A snarl *(1 mark)*

Poor smile *(1 mark)*

Looks sad *(1 mark)*

Unable to whistle *(1 mark)*

Drooping mouth *(1 mark)*

c *(1 mark for each correct answer, maximum 2 marks)* /2

Ptosis – worsens if you ask the patient to keep
looking up *(1 mark)*

Ophthalmoplegia *(1 mark)*

Diplopia *(1 mark)*

d *(1 mark for each correct answer, maximum 2 marks)* /2

Acetylcholine receptor antibodies can be found
in 90% of cases of myasthenia gravis *(1 mark)*

The Tensilon test – 10 mg IV edrophonium,
a short-acting anticholinesterase. A positive test
is when there is a rapid improvement in the
weakness *(1 mark)*

Nerve stimulation of a motor nerve shows a
decreased in evoked potential *(1 mark)*

Mediastinal imaging, either CT or MRI, to look
for a thymoma *(1 mark)*

e *(1 mark for each correct answer, maximum 3 marks)* /3

Anticholinesterase medication – neostigmine *(1 mark)*

Corticosteroids *(1 mark)*

Immunosuppressant medication – azathioprine
(1 mark)

Plasmaphoresis – this involves routing the person's
blood supply through a machine to remove the
harmful antibody-containing plasma from the blood
and replacing it with antibody-free plasma *(1 mark)*

Avoid triggers for attacks such as stress, infections
and becoming overtired *(1 mark)*

Summary

The cause of myasthenia gravis is not clearly known. Serum IgG antibodies to acetylcholine receptors have been found in the postsynaptic membrane of the neuromuscular junction. This leads to receptor loss, which is responsible for fatiguability encountered by patients. Some other causes of muscle fatiguability are polymyositis and SLE, so a full vasculitis screen is required to differentiate between these.

5 Renal Medicine and Urology

QUESTIONS

1 Stuart, a 17-year-old boy, awoke this morning with severe left flank pain, radiating to his groin. He has vomited on three occasions this morning. He has passed some urine, which he says appeared normal to him.

  a Give the two most likely diagnoses.   *2 marks*

  b On further questioning he tells you that the pain comes and goes every 5 minutes, and is the worst pain he has ever felt. He has also had pain when passing urine. Give two immediate investigations you would request in this case.   *2 marks*

  c Give two investigations you may wish to request on an outpatient basis.   *2 marks*

  d Outline four steps in your management of this patient.   *4 marks*

  e Give three common types of calculi.   *3 marks*

2 Sarah, a 29-year-old girl, has been brought into A & E with right flank pain, fever, and rigors. She has also been vomiting this morning, and feels generally unwell. She has recently had a course of trimethoprim from her GP.

  a What is the most likely diagnosis?   *1 mark*

  b State three blood tests you would request, and what might they show?   *3 marks*

  c Give two other tests you would ask for apart from imaging.   *2 marks*

  d Give three steps in your management of this condition.   *3 marks*

  e Give two possible complications of this condition.   *2 marks*

Complete SAQs for Medical Finals By P. Stather et al, Published 2010 by Blackwell Publishing, ISBN: 978-1-4501-8928-6.

3 Sheila, a 73-year-old lady, has come to see you in clinic complaining of a burning sensation when passing urine, and she says that her urine smells funny. She says this has not happened before, and she has no abdominal pain, and has not passed any blood.

  a Give three abnormalities you would expect to
find on a urine dip in this patient.   *3 marks*

  b Identify the three antibiotics commonly used to
treat a UTI in the community.   *3 marks*

  c State three pieces of advice you would give this
lady to prevent further UTIs.   *3 marks*

  d If this infection had occurred in a 3-year-old boy,
what two further investigations would you
request?   *2 marks*

4 Julie, a 27-year-old lady, has been admitted with complications of polycystic kidney disease. She has been monitored for this since she was a child as her mother had the same condition.

  a What is the usual genetic inheritance of this
condition?   *1 mark*

  b Suggest two of the likely symptoms that she is
suffering from.   *2 marks*

  c Name two imaging modalities you may use to
diagnose this condition.   *2 marks*

  d Give two features of your long-term management
of this patient.   *2 marks*

  e Give two problems that may occur in the future.   *2 marks*

  f Name one other place where cysts may occur in
any patient with this condition.   *1 mark*

5 Aseem, a 3-year-old boy, is brought to see you by his parents. They say that his face appears swollen, and he has gained a lot of weight recently. He has also been off his food. They have also noticed whilst potty training that his urine appears frothy, and he has had several UTIs in the past.

  a What is the diagnosis?   *1 mark*

  b What abnormality would you find on urine dip?   *1 mark*

  c You take a renal biopsy, which is sent for
investigations. What would you expect to see
on light microscopy of the sample?   *1 mark*

  d What would you see on electron microscopy?   *1 mark*

  e Give two treatment options for this condition.   *2 marks*

  f What is the usual progression of the disease?   *2 marks*

g Give two complications which may occur if
this is left untreated.   *2 marks*

6 Claire, a 35-year-old lady, has come to see you in the GP surgery
with a sore throat and cough, which has lasted for a week. She
has not had any rhinitis, although recalls that her son recently
had a cold.

a List four of the signs of pneumonia on examination
of the chest.   *4 marks*

Her examination is normal and you reassure her
and advise her to drink plenty of fluids. She returns
to see you in 10 days' time as she has noticed blood
in her urine, and her sore throat remains.
You suspect she may have post-streptococcal
glomerulonephritis.

b Give two other signs or symptoms of this condition.   *2 marks*
c Explain the pathophysiology behind this condition.   *2 marks*
d Give two complications of a kidney biopsy.   *2 marks*
e Give two possible long-term complications
of post-streptococcal glomerulonephritis.   *2 marks*

7 Patricia, a 72-year-old lady, has been admitted with collapse.
She was found at home by her carer, and was responsive, but
confused. You dip her urine which shows markers of a UTI, and
take some blood.

a Her blood tests come back showing her
inflammatory markers are raised. You also sent
a sample for U+E, which shows she is in renal
failure, with her previous U+E from 2 weeks ago
being normal. Give two features of the U+Es
which indicate renal failure.   *2 marks*
b What are the three categories of acute renal
failure, and give two common examples of each.   *6 marks*
c Outline five aspects of your management of
this patient.   *5 marks*

8 Abdel, a 75-year-old gentleman, is known to have type 1 diabetes. He undergoes regular monitoring for this, and his renal
function has been declining in recent months. He has not
noticed any other diabetic complications.

a Give four other things you monitor in
diabetic patients.   *4 marks*

b Name three risk factors other than diabetes for
developing chronic renal failure. *3 marks*

c List three symptoms of chronic renal failure. *3 marks*

d Abdel also has his blood pressure checked, which
is 170/105. Explain the pathophysiology behind
his hypertension. *3 marks*

e Abdel also suffers from anaemia. Explain the
cause of this. *1 mark*

9 Peter, a 63-year-old man, has just been diagnosed with chronic
renal failure secondary to type 2 diabetes. He is put on the
transplant list, and advised about renal replacement therapy.

a Give three advantages of haemodialysis and
three advantages of continuous ambulatory
peritoneal dialysis. *3 marks*

b Fortunately Peter has a son with matching tissue
type, who donates his kidney. What class of
medications will Peter need to take now? *1 mark*

c Give two common side effects of these medications. *2 marks*

d Apart from living related donors, give three other
sources of transplants for any organ. *3 marks*

e Suggest two problems that may occur with this
transplant. *2 marks*

f What advice should you give Peter's son after
the operation? *1 mark*

10 George, a 69-year-old man, comes to see you as he has noticed
blood in his urine. He has no past history of renal disease.

a Give two risk factors for developing
bladder cancer. *2 marks*

b How is a diagnosis of bladder cancer made? *1 mark*

c His tumour is staged at T1 N0 M0. What
treatment would be most appropriate in his case? *2 marks*

d George moves abroad, and unfortunately is lost to
follow-up. He presents 5 years later with more
haematuria. Investigations are repeated which
show enlargement of the tumour, which is now
T4 N1 M0. What does T4 correspond to
anatomically in relation to bladder tumours? *2 marks*

e What two further treatment options may be
available? *2 marks*

f George presents later on in acute renal failure.
What is likely to be the cause? *2 marks*

11 Paul, a 76-year-old man, has noticed that he has to urinate more frequently in recent months, including 3–4 times at night. He is also finding it difficult to urinate, with some dribbling after he has finished.

   a What are the two most likely differential diagnoses? *2 marks*

   b What features might help you to differentiate between these two conditions on PR examination? *2 marks*

   c Name one other test which may be performed to differentiate between these diagnoses. *1 mark*

   d The above tests lead you to believe that the diagnosis is malignant. Give two treatment options available. *2 marks*

   e Paul presents in 2 years' time with lower back pain. What are you concerned about, and what can be done about this? *2 marks*

   f Paul goes into urinary retention. Give two immediate options available to treat this. *2 marks*

   g If the diagnosis wasn't malignant, suggest two medications which could be used to relieve his symptoms, and how they work. *2 marks*

12 Kim, a 57-year-old sales assistant, presents to the GP surgery with frank haematuria. This has not happened before, and she is complaining of no pain, although she says she has recently had several nose bleeds, and is being investigated for swollen joints.

   a Name four different sites which may be causing the haematuria, with two common examples for each. *4 marks*

   b Give two other causes of red urine, which is not due to blood. *2 marks*

   c Following this history you do several investigations, including a vasculitic screen, which show that she is suffering from Wegener's granulomatosis. Name one abnormality you may see on CXR of a patient with Wegener's. *1 mark*

   d What test is typically positive in this condition? *1 mark*

   e Name two medications you would use to treat this condition. *2 marks*

   f Following your treatment her symptoms settle, and she improves. What will you tell her with regard to her long-term management and prognosis? *2 marks*

Renal Medicine and Urology

ANSWERS

1 a *(1 mark for each correct answer, maximum 2 marks)*   `/2`
Kidney stone *(1 mark)*
Testicular torsion *(1 mark)*
Pyelonephritis *(1 mark)*
  b Urine dip – blood *(1 mark)*   `/2`
Renal imaging (KUB, IVU, ultrasound,
    or CT) – showing stones *(1 mark)*
  c Measure calcium, oxalate and uric acid levels in the   `/2`
blood and urine *(1 mark)*
24-hour urine collection for volume *(1 mark)*
  d Analgesia *(1 mark)*   `/4`
IV fluids *(1 mark)*
If the stone doesn't pass by itself then lithotripsy
    may be required *(1 mark)*
Give the patient advice regarding fluid intake *(1 mark)*
  e *(1 mark for each correct answer, maximum 3 marks)*   `/3`
Calcium oxalate *(1 mark)*
Calcium phosphate *(1 mark)*
Uric acid *(1 mark)*
Cysteine *(1 mark)*

Summary

Renal calculi occur in 2% of the population, with the majority having a recurrence within 5 years. 90% are radio-opaque and can be detected on x-ray. Stones form due to urinary stasis due to a poor urine output, or obstruction. Stones may also be due to an altered urinary pH, low citrate concentrations (as citrate inhibits stone formation), infection, and hypercalciuria or hyperoxaluria.

2 a Pyelonephritis *(1 mark)*   `/1`
  b FBC – high WCC and neutrophils *(1 mark)*   `/3`
CRP – raised inflammatory marker indicative
    of infection *(1 mark)*

U+E – urea and creatinine will be raised if any
renal impairment *(1 mark)*

c Urine dip and culture *(1 mark)* `/2`
Blood culture *(1 mark)*

d *(1 mark for each correct answer, maximum 3 marks)* `/3`
Analgesia *(1 mark)*
IV fluids *(1 mark)*
IV antibiotics *(1 mark)*
Monitor renal function *(1 mark)*

e *(1 mark for each correct answer, maximum 2 marks)* `/2`
Acute renal failure *(1 mark)*
Sepsis *(1 mark)*
Perinephric abscess *(1 mark)*
Recurrence of pyelonephritis *(1 mark)*

Summary

Pyelonephritis is a serious infection, often causing sepsis. Patients present with systemic symptoms such as fever, rigors, loin pain and tenderness, nausea, vomiting, and hypotension or shock, possibly with the symptoms of a lower urinary tract infection. Treatment should be instigated rapidly to prevent deterioration of renal function by giving IV fluids, and treating the infection with IV antibiotics.

3 a *(1 mark for each correct answer, maximum 3 marks)* `/3`
Presence of leukocytes *(1 mark)*
Presence of nitrites *(1 mark)*
Presence of blood *(1 mark)*
Presence of protein *(1 mark)*

b Trimethoprim *(1 mark)* `/3`
Nitrofurantoin *(1 mark)*
Amoxicillin *(1 mark)*

c *(1 mark for each correct answer, maximum 3 marks)* `/3`
Wipe from front to back *(1 mark)*
Wear cotton undergarments *(1 mark)*
Urinate after intercourse *(1 mark)*
Keep the genital area clean *(1 mark)*
Drink plenty of fluids *(1 mark)*
Drink cranberry juice *(1 mark)*

d Ultrasound of the kidneys *(1 mark)* `/2`
Voiding cystourethrogram *(1 mark)*

Summary
UTIs are more common in women due to their shorter urethra. *E. coli* accounts for 85% of UTIs although *Klebsiella, Proteus* and *Streptococcus faecalis* infection may also occur. There are several underlying predisposing factors, such as diabetes, analgesic nephropathy, immunodeficiency, renal calculi, urinary obstruction, vesicoureteric reflux, PUJ obstruction, catheterisation, incomplete voiding, urinary stasis and pregnancy.

4 a Autosomal dominant *(1 mark)* ⬜ /1
  b *(1 mark for each correct answer, maximum 2 marks)* ⬜ /2
    Abdominal pain *(1 mark)*
    Flank pain which may be bilateral *(1 mark)*
    Nocturia *(1 mark)*
    Haematuria *(1 mark)*
    Drowsiness *(1 mark)*
    Joint pain *(1 mark)*
  c *(1 mark for each correct answer, maximum 2 marks)* ⬜ /2
    Ultrasound *(1 mark)*
    CT *(1 mark)*
    MRI *(1 mark)*
    IVP *(1 mark)*
  d *(1 mark for each correct answer, maximum 2 marks)* ⬜ /2
    Antihypertensives *(1 mark)*
    Diuretics *(1 mark)*
    Low salt diet *(1 mark)*
    Prompt treatment of UTIs *(1 mark)*
    Consider for renal transplant *(1 mark)*
  e *(1 mark for each correct answer, maximum 2 marks)* ⬜ /2
    Hypertension *(1 mark)*
    Recurrent kidney infections *(1 mark)*
    Chronic renal failure *(1 mark)*
    Anaemia *(1 mark)*
    Liver failure *(1 mark)*
  f *(maximum 1 mark)* ⬜ /1
    Liver *(1 mark)*
    Pancreas *(1 mark)*
    Testes *(1 mark)*

Summary
Polycystic kidney disease is most commonly due to a genetic defect on the long arm of chromosome 16, although in 10–15% of

patients is due to a defect in chromosome 4. It accounts for roughly 5–10% of patients on renal dialysis.

5 a Minimal change glomerulonephritis *(1 mark)* ☐ /1
  b Presence of protein *(1 mark)* ☐ /1
  c Nothing *(1 mark)* ☐ /1
  d Fusion of the podocytes (epithelial cell foot ☐ /1
    processes) *(1 mark)*
  e *(1 mark for each correct answer, maximum 2 marks)* ☐ /2
    Prednisolone *(1 mark)*
    Cyclophosphamide *(1 mark)*
    Cyclosporin *(1 mark)*
    Azathioprine *(1 mark)*
    ACE inhibitors *(1 mark)* – reduce proteinuria
  f Tends to resolve following a course of steroids, ☐ /2
    however a small percentage have recurrent
    episodes *(1 mark)*
    It does not cause end-stage renal failure *(1 mark)*
  g *(1 mark for each correct answer, maximum 2 marks)* ☐ /2
    Heavy proteinuria may over time lead to muscle
    wasting *(1 mark)*
    Thinning of skin *(1 mark)*
    Growth failure *(1 mark)*

Summary

Minimal change glomerulonephritis has two peaks of incidence, initially at 2 years, then 40. The majority of causes are idiopathic, although it can also be due to drugs such as NSAIDs, interferon and penicillin, toxins such as mercury, lithium and bee stings, infections such as HIV and immunisations, tumours such as Hodgkin's lymphoma, and carcinomas, and post-haematopoietic stem cell transplant.

6 a *(1 mark for each correct answer, maximum 4 marks)* ☐ /4
    Decreased chest expansion *(1 mark)*
    Decreased air entry *(1 mark)*
    Dullness to percussion *(1 mark)*
    Crepitations *(1 mark)*
    Vocal fremitus/resonance *(1 mark)*
    Her examination is normal and you reassure her
    and advise her to drink plenty of fluids. She
    returns to see you in 10 days' time as she has

noticed blood in her urine, and her sore throat remains. You suspect she may have post-streptococcal glomerulonephritis.

b *(1 mark for each correct answer, maximum 2 marks)*   `/2`
Decreased urine output *(1 mark)*
Oedema *(1 mark)*
Rust coloured urine *(1 mark)*
Joint pain or stiffness *(1 mark)*

c Infection with group A haemolytic streptococcus   `/2`
causes inflammation in the glomeruli *(1 mark)*,
so the kidneys are unable to filter the blood
sufficiently and blood leaks through the
glomeruli *(1 mark)*

d *(1 mark for each correct answer, maximum 2 marks)*   `/2`
Haematuria *(1 mark)*
Haematoma formation *(1 mark)*
Infection *(1 mark)*
Arteriovenous fistula *(1 mark)*

e *(1 mark for each correct answer, maximum 2 marks)*   `/2`
Acute renal failure *(1 mark)*
Chronic renal failure *(1 mark)*
Congestive heart failure *(1 mark)*
Nephrotic syndrome *(1 mark)*

Summary

Post-streptococcal glomerulonephritis usually occurs in children 1–3 weeks following a streptococcal infection of the pharynx, otitis media, or cellulitis. There is no proven treatment for the condition, and recovery is usually spontaneous. Management is to reduce any oedema with furosemide, treat any uraemia, possibly with dialysis, and monitor for hypertensive encephalopathy.

7 a *(1 mark for each correct answer, maximum 2 marks)*   `/2`
Raised urea *(1 mark)*
High potassium *(1 mark)*
Raised creatinine *(1 mark)*
Low eGFR *(1 mark)*

b Pre-renal *(1 mark)* – poor blood supply to kidney   `/6`
due to hypotension, caused by trauma, surgery,
septic shock, haemorrhage, burns, or dehydration
(1 mark for each example, maximum 2 marks)

Renal *(1 mark)* – pyelonephritis, septicaemia, glomerulonephritis, toxins, haemolyisis, multiple myeloma
(1 mark for each example, maximum 2 marks)

Post renal *(1 mark)* – obstruction to the urinary flow,
bilateral kidney stones, prostatic enlargement, bladder cancer obstructing flow *(1 mark for each example,
maximum 2 marks)*

c *(1 mark for each correct answer, maximum 5 marks)*   /5

Send urine for culture and sensitivities *(1 mark)*
Antibiotics for UTI *(1 mark)*
Catheterise *(1 mark)*
IV fluids *(1 mark)*
Fluid balance and daily weights *(1 mark)*
Stop nephrotoxic medications *(1 mark)*
Daily U+Es to monitor renal function and
    potassium *(1 mark)*
Renal review if no improvement *(1 mark)*

Summary

The typical presenting features of acute renal failure are oliguria,
anorexia, nausea, vomiting, drowsiness, apathy, confusion, muscle
twitching, fits and coma.

Management is by identifying and correcting the underlying
cause. In pre-renal failure, rapid treatment may prevent acute
tubular necrosis. This is done by giving loop diuretics along with
IV fluids, and stopping any nephrotoxic drugs. If the cause is a urinary tract obstruction then catheterisation should be done. Renal
causes require rapid treatment of the underlying condition.

8 a *(1 mark for each correct answer, maximum 4 marks)*   /4

Feet (1 mark)
Eyes *(1 mark)*
Lipids *(1 mark)*
Blood pressure *(1 mark)*
Glucose levels *(1 mark)*
HbA1c *(1 mark)*

b *(1 mark for each correct answer, maximum 3 marks)*   /3

Age *(1 mark)*
Race *(1 mark)*
Smoking *(1 mark)*
Hypertension *(1 mark)*

Family History *(1 mark)*
Underlying chronic renal diseases such as
glomerulonephritis or PCKD *(1 mark)*

c *(1 mark for each correct answer, maximum 3 marks)* ☐ /3
Hiccups *(1 mark)*
Fatigue *(1 mark)*
Pruritis *(1 mark)*
Headache *(1 mark)*
Weight loss and loss of appetite *(1 mark)*
Nausea and vomiting *(1 mark)*
Bruising *(1 mark)*
Lethargy *(1 mark)*
Malaise *(1 mark)*
Palpitations *(1 mark)*
Breathlessness *(1 mark)*
Oedema *(1 mark)*
Chest pain due to pericarditis *(1 mark)*

d *(1 mark for each correct answer, maximum 3 marks)* ☐ /3
Decreased kidney perfusion causes increased
production of renin *(1 mark)*, which in turn
increases aldosterone and angiotensin levels
(1 mark) causing vasoconstriction *(1 mark)*. They
also increase sodium and fluid retention *(1 mark)*.

e Erythropoietin production from the kidneys is ☐ /1
decreased. *(1 mark)*

Summary

Chronic renal failure is an irreversible deterioration in renal function, which develops over a period of years. It initially manifests as a biochemical abnormality, progressing to loss of excretory, metabolic and endocrine functions. Symptoms generally do not develop until 75% of the renal function is lost.

9 a Haemodialysis – no need for peritoneal tube so ☐ /3
lower infection risk, treatment in hospital so
regular monitoring, treatment can be altered
easily, increased freedom on days when no
dialysis needed *(½ mark for each answer,
maximum 1½ marks)*
Continuous ambulatory peritoneal dialysis – lower
cost, can be done at home so more freedom, easier

BP control, preserves residual renal function for longer, blood sugar control improved
(*½ mark for each answer, maximum 1½ marks*)

b Immunosuppressants *(1 mark)* – the typical regime is prednisolone, tacrolimus and mycophenolate `/1`

c *(1 mark for each correct answer, maximum 2 marks)* `/2`
Infection *(1 mark)*
Skin cancer *(1 mark)*
Kaposi's sarcoma *(1 mark)*
Lymphoma *(1 mark)*
Cardiac damage *(1 mark)*
Increased risk of sunburn *(1 mark)*

d *(1 mark for each correct answer, maximum 3 marks)* `/3`
Cadaver donors *(1 mark)*
Living emotionally related donors *(1 mark)*
Living non-related donor *(1 mark)*
Xenograft *(1 mark)*

e *(1 mark for each correct answer, maximum 2 marks)* `/2`
Rejection *(1 mark)*
Infection *(1 mark)*
Failure of the donor kidney *(1 mark)*

f There is no evidence to suggest that Peter is at an increased risk of renal failure, and he is free to live a normal healthy lifestyle, with no extra limitations *(1 mark)*. The average lifespan for people who donate is higher than average due to the thorough screening prior to donation, ensuring that only those in good health may donate. `/1`

Summary

Haemodialysis is where blood is pumped across one surface of a semi-permeable membrane whilst an osmotically balanced solution of electrolytes, buffer and glucose in water flows across the other surface.

CAPD requires a peritoneal membrane and blood flow. This involves putting dialysis fluid into the peritoneum, and leaving it there for several hours, during which the patient is free to move. The fluid is then drained out and replaced. The patient usually undergoes 4 × 2 litre exchanges per day.

10 a *(1 mark for each correct answer, maximum 2 marks)* `/2`
Working in the chemical, cable, or rubber industries *(1 mark)*
Smoking *(1 mark)*
Exposure to drugs such as phenacetin and cyclophosphamide *(1 mark)*
Exposure to aniline dyes *(1 mark)*
Chronic inflammation such as schistosomiasis or bladder stone *(1 mark)*

b Cystoscopy and biopsy *(1 mark)* `/1`

c *(1 mark for each correct answer, maximum 2 marks)* `/2`
Local cystodiathermy or resection *(1 mark)*
Regular recheck cystocopies *(1 mark)*
Regular cytological examination of urine *(1 mark)*
George moves abroad, and unfortunately is lost to follow-up. He presents 5 years later with more haematuria. Investigations are repeated which show enlargement of the tumour, which is now T4 N1 M0.

d The cancer has spread through the bladder endothelium, mucosa and muscular wall *(1 mark)* and into the surrounding tissues *(1 mark)* `/2`

e Intravesical chemotherapy *(1 mark)* `/2`
Total cystectomy and radiotherapy for metastases *(1 mark)*

f Extension of the tumour causing blockage of urinary flow *(1 mark)*, leading to post renal failure due to obstruction *(1 mark)* `/2`

Summary

Bladder cancer is commonly a transitional cell carcinoma. Localised bladder tumours may be treated with diathermy and followed up with cystoscopy. Extensive superficial tumours of the bladder may be treated with intravesical chemotherapy. A total cystectomy can be performed if there are severe symptoms, and metastases can be treated with chemotherapy or radiotherapy.

11 a Benign prostatic hypertrophy *(1 mark)* `/2`
Prostate cancer *(1 mark)*

b BPH – smooth *(1 mark)* `/2`
Cancer – hard and irregular *(1 mark)*

c *(1 mark for each correct answer, maximum 2 marks)* /1
Prostatic specific antigen *(1 mark)*
Biopsy *(1 mark)*

d *(1 mark for each correct answer, maximum 2 marks)* /2
Radical prostatectomy *(1 mark)*
Radiotherapy via external beam *(1 mark)*
Brachiotherapy *(1 mark)*
Observation and symptomatic relief such as TURP
    (1 mark)
LHRH antagonists *(1 mark)*

e *(1 mark for each correct answer, maximum 2 marks)* /2
Metastatic spread to the bone *(1 mark)*
Palliative radiotherapy and pain relief *(1 mark)*
Hormonal therapy *(1 mark)*

f Urethral catheterisation *(1 mark)* /2
Suprapubic catheterisation *(1 mark)*

g *(1 mark for each correct answer, maximum 2 marks)* /2
Anti-androgens such as finasteride *(1 mark)* –
    decreases hormones produced by the prostate,
    therefore decreasing its size, however may cause
    decreased libido and impotence
Alpha-1 blockers *(1 mark)* – relax the bladder neck
Antibiotics *(1 mark)* – to treat chronic prostatitis

Summary

Prostate cancer is the second commonest malignancy in men, occurring in 80% of men over 80 years. Most are adenocarcinomas, and may spread to bone, seminal vesicles, the bladder or the rectum. It is often asymptomatic, but can cause nocturia, hesitancy, poor stream, terminal dribbling and urinary obstruction. Weight loss and bone pain are indicative of metastases. Prostate cancer is often controlled with hormone suppressive therapy, and many men will live for years even when diagnosed with metastatic disease.

12 a *(maximum 4 marks)* /4
Kidneys – infection, glomerulonephritis, tumour,
    polycystic kidney disease, trauma, interstitial
    nephritis *(1 mark for site and any 2 examples)*
Ureters – trauma, tumour, stones *(1 mark for site and
    any 2 examples)*

Bladder – infection, tumour, trauma, stones
(1 mark for site and any 2 examples)
Urethra – trauma, stones, tumours, foreign bodies
(1 mark for site and any 2 examples)
Systemic conditions – clotting disorders,
thrombocytopenia, vascilitis, endocarditis,
sickle cell *(1 mark for site and any 2 examples)*
Other sites – fistulae or inflammation in adjacent
organs such as the colon, diverticulitis,
inflammatory bowel disease, PID, appendicitis,
or carcinoma of the colon *(½ mark for 1 example)*

b *(1 mark for each correct answer, maximum 2 marks)* `/2`
Beetroot *(1 mark)*
Medications such as rifampicin *(1 mark)*
Pigmentation from haemolysis and rhabdomyolysis
(1 mark)

c *(maximum 1 mark)* `/1`
Nodules *(1 mark)*
Infiltrates *(1 mark)*
Cavities *(1 mark)*

d c-ANCA *(1 mark)* `/1`

e *(1 mark for each correct answer, maximum 2 marks)* `/2`
Prednisolone *(1 mark)*
Cyclophosphamide *(1 mark)*
Azathioprine *(1 mark)*
Methotrexate *(1 mark)*

f *(1 mark for each correct answer, maximum 2 marks)* `/2`
She will remain on lifelong medications *(1 mark)*
There is a high chance of relapse in the future
(1 mark)
Regular blood test monitoring should be done
of inflammatory markers and c-ANCA *(1 mark)*

Summary

There are several causes of haematuria, however it is most important to rule out any underlying neoplastic cause before coming to any other diagnosis. Haematuria must be distinguished as to whether it is throughout voiding, or principally at the beginning or end of each void, as this guides us towards the likely part of the urinary tract it is coming from, and therefore the likely diagnosis.

6 Endocrinology

QUESTIONS

1 Alice, a 55-year-old lady, comes to see you in your GP surgery complaining of a tremor. She has also noticed that she has lost weight recently, is finding it difficult to concentrate, and appears to be losing her hair.

   a What is the most likely diagnosis?   *1 mark*
   b List three other common causes of a tremor.   *3 marks*
   c Give four other symptoms this lady may have.   *2 marks*
   d What would you expect her TFTs to show?   *2 marks*
   e Give two treatment options which are available
   for this condition.   *2 marks*

2 Bethany, a 46-year-old lady, attends your GP surgery saying that she has been feeling low for the past few months. She has also noticed that her skin has become poor, and she has been gaining weight, despite dieting.

   a What is the most likely diagnosis?   *1 mark*
   b Give two other symptoms she may have noticed.   *2 marks*
   c State two further signs you might elicit on
   examination.   *2 marks*
   d What is the treatment for Bethany's condition?   *1 mark*
   e What is a potential complication of this treatment?   *1 mark*
   f What is the serious, potential complication of
   this condition if left untreated?   *1 mark*
   g Give two signs or symptoms of this complication.   *2 marks*

3 Andrew, a 42-year-old gentleman, has been gaining weight for the past year, particularly around his abdomen, and his wife has said that his face in particular looks fat, with poor skin, and increased facial hair. They are both confused as to why this has

Complete SAQs for Medical Finals By P. Stather et al, Published 2010 by Blackwell Publishing, ISBN: 978-1-4501-8928-6.

happened, as he does not drink alcohol, and has a reasonably good diet. He is on no medication at present.

a Give three more signs or symptoms you may find. *3 marks*

b What is the biochemical cause of this condition? *1 mark*

c Give two tests you would request to determine
that this was the cause. *2 marks*

d Which two further radiological investigations
would you request to determine the cause of the
condition and why? *2 marks*

e Give two further complications he is at risk of. *2 marks*

4 Bernard, a 50-year-old man, has been diagnosed with Addison's disease.

a Name two of the hormones involved in Addison's
disease. *2 marks*

b Where are these hormones produced? *1 mark*

c Give three symptoms of Addison's disease. *3 marks*

d Give four investigations that you would request
for this patient. *4 marks*

e What is the treatment for Addison's disease? *2 marks*

5 Cynthia, a 60-year-old lady, attends her GP surgery for a routine physical, during which bloods are taken. Her glucose comes back at 9.1, and you ask her to return to your surgery.

a What would be your next step in her management? *1 mark*

b This test confirms a diagnosis of type 2 diabetes.
Give two possible drug treatments for this lady. *2 marks*

c What three pieces of advice would you give her
regarding her lifestyle? *3 marks*

d Which three other systems will need regular
monitoring following her diagnosis? *3 marks*

e This lady develops a blood pressure of 160/95. What
should her blood pressure ideally be controlled at? *1 mark*

f Which class of antihypertensive medications
should you ideally prescribe for her, and why? *2 marks*

6 Carl, a 13-year-old boy, who comes to see you with his mother, has noticed that he appears to be drinking excessively, and is passing a large amount of urine. He has also lost weight recently.

a What is the most likely diagnosis? *1 mark*

b Suggest two tests you would perform to make
this diagnosis. *2 marks*

c What three different types of subcutaneous insulin
are there? *3 marks*

d Carl is started on insulin and presents to A & E a
few weeks later having been unrousable from bed
that morning. What is the likely diagnosis and how
would you confirm this?   *2 marks*

e Give three ways in which this could be prevented
in the future.   *3 marks*

7 Anne, a 9-year-old girl, with no past medical history, is brought
into the A & E department by her parents who are very concerned. She has had a decreased conscious level this morning,
and her breathing has been rapid, with abdominal pain.

a Give three immediate investigations you would
carry out.   *3 marks*

b Give three aspects of the immediate management
for this patient.   *3 marks*

This patients ABGs are done, and come back with
the following results:

pH	–	7.3
pO_2	–	12.1
pCO_2	–	4.3
HCO_3	–	18
Base excess	–	-3.1

c What is the interpretation of these results?   *2 marks*

d What is the metabolic process behind this patient
becoming ill?   *3 marks*

8 Charles, a 62-year-old man, comes to see you in your GP surgery. His wife has noticed that his appearance has changed
recently, and he has noticed that his shoe size has increased
from a 9 to a 10 over the past 2 years, and he has had to buy
new gloves, as his old pair became tight.

a What is the likely diagnosis?   *1 mark*

b What is the hormonal abnormality in this
condition, and from which gland does it arise?   *2 marks*

c Name three other hormones secreted by this gland.   *3 marks*

d Give four other signs or symptoms you would
look for in this patient.   *4 marks*

e Give three further long-term complications you
would monitor for in this patient.   *3 marks*

9 Carla, a 60-year-old lady, is admitted to the psychiatric unit
with severe depression. Her routine bloods are sent, and she is
started on an antidepressant.

a Which group of antidepressants would you start
her on first, and give one example.   *2 marks*

b Her blood tests come back showing a raised
calcium level. What is the most common
endocrine cause of hypercalcaemia? *1 mark*

c Give three symptoms of hypercalcaemia. *3 marks*

d Suggest three aspects of the treatment you
would give for her hypercalcaemia in the
short term. *3 marks*

e What will be required in the long term to treat
the underlying cause? *1 mark*

f Vitamin D is important in calcium homeostasis.
Explain the three ways in which this works. *3 marks*

10 Alison, a 36-year-old lady, comes to see you as she is having
palpitations. On examination you find her BP 190/115, which
is confirmed on repeat. She has no family history of note, and
the rest of her examination is normal.

a Give three causes of secondary hypertension. *3 marks*

b The only abnormality found on investigation is
a raised plasma catecholamine, which is
confirmed with a 24-hour urine sample. What
diagnosis is this consistent with? *1 mark*

c Explain the biochemical basis for these symptoms. *3 marks*

d Apart from palpitations, give three other
symptoms that may occur in this condition. *3 marks*

e What two medications would you use to control
the blood pressure in this patient? *2 marks*

f What is the surgical management of this patient? *1 mark*

11 Brenda, a 27-year-old lady, comes to see you with her husband
in the GP surgery. She has been having galactorrhoea for the
past 2 weeks, and on further history says that her and her husband have been trying for a baby for the past year, with no success. You suspect a prolactinoma.

a List three other symptoms she may have. *3 marks*

b From where does a prolactinoma arise? *2 marks*

c What two tests or investigations would you
request to diagnose this condition? *2 marks*

d Give two different examples of treatment
available for this lady. *2 marks*

e If this tumour is left untreated and grows,
what visual abnormality may arise and why? *2 marks*

Endocrinology

ANSWERS

1 a Hyperthyroidism *(1 mark)* `/1`
  b *(1 mark for each correct answer, maximum 3 marks)* `/3`
   Benign essential tremor *(1 mark)*
   Substance withdrawal *(1 mark)*
   Parkinson's *(1 mark)*
   Anxiety *(1 mark)*
   Iatrogenic *(1 mark)*
  c *(1 mark for each correct answer, maximum 2 marks)* `/2`
   Sweating *(1 mark)*
   Palpitations *(1 mark)*
   Fatigue *(1 mark)*
   Heat intolerance *(1 mark)*
   Diarrhoea *(1 mark)*
   Amenorrhoea *(1 mark)*
  d TSH low *(1 mark)* `/2`
   T3/T4 high *(1 mark)*
  e *(1 mark for each correct answer, maximum 2 marks)* `/2`
   Radioactive iodine therapy *(1 mark)*
   Thyroidectomy (partial or total) *(1 mark)*
   Carbimazole *(1 mark)*
   Propylthiouracil *(1 mark)*

Summary

Hyperthyroidism affects 1/50 females and 1/250 males. it is due to an excess of T3 and T4 causing thyrotoxicosis. An acute exacerbation of symptoms is called a thyrotoxic crisis, usually brought on by infection. diagnosis is by measuring TSH, free T3 and free T4. Raised TSH suggests the fault is in the pituitary or hypothalamus, whereas low TSH is due to a thyroid problem.

2 a Hypothyroidism *(1 mark)* `/1`
  b *(1 mark for each correct answer, maximum 2 marks)* `/2`
   Heavy irregular periods *(1 mark)*

Cold intolerance *(1 mark)*
Constipation *(1 mark)*
Hoarse voice *(1 mark)*
c *(1 mark for each correct answer, maximum 2 marks)* `/2`
Slowed reflexes *(1 mark)*
Goitre *(1 mark)*
Hair loss *(1 mark)*
Oedema *(1 mark)*
Loss of outer third of eyebrows *(1 mark)*
d Thyroxine *(1 mark)* `/1`
e Hyperthyroidism *(1 mark)* `/1`
f Myxoedema coma *(1 mark)* `/1`
g *(1 mark for each correct answer, maximum 2 marks)* `/2`
Unresponsiveness *(1 mark)*
Decreased respiratory rate *(1 mark)*
Low BP *(1 mark)*
Low glucose *(1 mark)*
Low temperature *(1 mark)*

Summary

Hypothyroidism affects 1/100 females and 1/500 males. It presents gradually with several symptoms, such as mental slowing, apathy, tiredness, psychosis, coarse thin hair, loss of the outer third of the eyebrows, myxoedema causing a pale puffy face, goitre, hoarse voice, bradycardia, slowing of muscle activity, proximal myopathy, constipation, amenorrhoea, cold hands, carpal tunnel, slow reflexes, weight gain, intolerance to cold, and decreased sweating. T3 and T4 levels are usually low, with a raised TSH, due to insensitivity of the thyroid, however if TSH is low then there is likely to be a hypothalamic or pituitary lesion.

3 a *(1 mark for each correct answer, maximum 3 marks)* `/3`
Thin skin *(1 mark)*
Easy bruising *(1 mark)*
Purple striae *(1 mark)*
Weakness *(1 mark)*
Buffalo hump *(1 mark)*
Impotence *(1 mark)*
b Raised cortisol levels *(1 mark)* `/1`
c *(1 mark for each correct answer, maximum 2 marks)* `/2`
Urine cortisol level *(1 mark)*
Dexamethasone suppression test *(1 mark)*

Serial serum cortisol levels (9 a.m. cortisol, levels peak in the morning and need to be measured at this time each day for validity) *(1 mark)*

d *(1 mark for each correct answer, maximum 2 marks)* `/2`
Cranial CT for pituitary tumour *(1 mark)*
Abdominal CT for adrenal tumour *(1 mark)*
CXR for tumour (bronchial carcinoma can secrete ACTH-like substance) *(1 mark)*

e *(1 mark for each correct answer, maximum 2 marks)* `/2`
Diabetes *(1 mark)*
Hypertension *(1 mark)*
Infections *(1 mark)*
Osteoporosis *(1 mark)*
Hypokalaemia *(1 mark)*
Kidney stones *(1 mark)*
Complications of enlargement of a pituitary tumour such as raised intracranial pressure *(1 mark)* or damage to the optic chiasm *(1 mark)*

Summary

Cushing's syndrome is an excess of glucocorticoids. Pituitary-dependant cortisol excess is Cushing's disease, caused by ectopic ACTH-secreting tumours such as bronchial carcinoma, small cell lung carcinoma, and pancreatic carcinoma.

The most common cause of Cushing's syndrome is iatrogenic, due to prolonged steroid use. Cushing's disease is the next commonest cause, accounting for about 80% of endogenous causes. Pituitary tumours are another cause, although these are usually microadenomas, so there are no other features of a pituitary mass.

4 a *(1 mark for each correct answer, maximum 2 marks)* `/2`
Cortisol *(1 mark)*
Aldosterone *(1 mark)*
Sex hormones *(1 mark)*
b Adrenal cortex *(1 mark)* `/1`
c *(1 mark for each correct answer, maximum 3 marks)* `/3`
Weakness *(1 mark)*
Fatigue *(1 mark)*
Vomiting *(1 mark)*
Dizziness due to low sodium causing hypotension *(1 mark)*
Weight loss *(1 mark)*
Poor appetite *(1 mark)*

Diarrhoea *(1 mark)*
Darkening of the skin (palmer creases) *(1 mark)*
Slow movements *(1 mark)*
Salt craving *(1 mark)*
d *(1 mark for each correct answer, maximum 4 marks)*   /4
U+E *(1 mark)*
Cortisol (9am) *(1 mark)*
ACTH *(1 mark)*
Aldosterone *(1 mark)*
Synacthen test (short or long) *(1 mark)*
BP *(1 mark)*
Abdominal x-ray/CT *(1 mark)*
e Hydrocortisone *(1 mark)* and fludrocortisone   /2
(1 mark) – both glucocorticoids and
mineralocorticoids need to be replaced.

Summary

Addison's disease is a rare condition with an incidence of 8 per million. It can be caused by primary adrenal hypofunction, due to autoimmune disease, TB, or bilateral adrenalectomy, or secondary causes such as hypothalamic or pituitary disease, or glucocorticoid therapy.

An Addisonian crisis is a critical condition due to loss of all adrenal function. The patient will be in circulatory shock with hyponatraemia, hyperkalaemia, and possibly hypoglycaemia. It is most commonly precipitated by surgery or infection. Management of an Addisonian crisis is with IV saline, glucocorticoids such as 8 mg intravenous dexamethasone, and dextrose if hypoglycaemic, then replacement of glucocorticoids with hydrocortisone, and monitoring therapy clinically.

5 a *(maximum 1 mark)*   /1
Fasting glucose *(1 mark)*
An oral glucose tolerance test *(1 mark)*
b *(1 mark for each correct answer, maximum 2 marks)*   /2
Biguanides – metformin *(1 mark)*
Sulphonylureas – gliclazide *(1 mark)*
Insulin *(1 mark)*
Thiazolidinediones *(1 mark)*
alpha glucosidase inhibitors *(1 mark)*
c *(1 mark for each correct answer, maximum 3 marks)*   /3
Reduce weight *(1 mark)*
Increase exercise *(1 mark)*
Stop smoking *(1 mark)*

Decrease alcohol *(1 mark)*
Low fat diet *(1 mark)*
More fruit and vegetables *(1 mark)*
d *(1 mark for each correct answer, maximum 3 marks)*   /3
Eyes *(1 mark)*
Feet *(1 mark)*
Kidneys *(1 mark)*
Cardiovascular *(1 mark)*
e 130/80 *(1 mark)*   /1
f ACE inhibitors (not as effective in Afro-Carribean   /2
ethnic groups) *(1 mark)*
They are proven to have extra benefits protecting
the kidneys in diabetic patients *(1 mark)*

Summary

Management of patients with diabetes is done as a preventive measure for future complications. Initially lifestyle modifications such as regular exercise, healthy diet, reducing alcohol consumption and cessation of smoking should be encouraged, followed by oral hypoglycaemic drugs such as sulfonylurea, biguanides, alpha-glucosidase inhibitors and thiazolidinediones. Insulin may also be needed in the long term. Therapeutic goals are to maintain glycaemic control and effective treatment of hypertension, which greatly reduces diabetic complications.

6 a Type 1 diabetes *(1 mark)*   /1
b *(1 mark for each correct answer, maximum 2 marks)*   /2
Random glucose level *(1 mark)*
Fasting glucose level *(1 mark)*
Oral glucose tolerance test *(1 mark)*
Check urine for ketones *(1 mark)*
c Short acting *(1 mark)*   /3
Medium acting *(1 mark)*
Long acting *(1 mark)*
d Hypoglycaemia *(1 mark)*   /2
BM sticks and random glucose test *(1 mark)*
e *(1 mark for each correct answer, maximum 3 marks)*   /3
Alter the insulin regime *(1 mark)*
Ensure meals are eaten regularly *(1 mark)*
Keep a sugary drink or snack by the bedside *(1 mark)*
Teach Carl the signs of a hypoglycaemic attack *(1 mark)*
Provide the parents with glucose gel *(1 mark)*

Refer Carl to the diabetes specialist nurse for support
and further information *(1 mark)*

Summary

Type 1 diabetes occurs partially due to genetics, which accounts
for roughly one-third of susceptibility, associated with HLA-DR3
and DR4, however environmental factors also have a role, as the
concordance rate in monozygotic twins is less than 40%. A variety of factors are implicated, including several viruses, diet such
as bovine serum albumin in cow's milk, stress, and immunological
factors causing a destruction of insulin-secreting cells over many
years. The classical presentation occurs when more than 90% of
cells are destroyed, so there is very little insulin production left.

7 a *(1 mark for each correct answer, maximum 3 marks)* ___/3___
BP *(1 mark)*
Pulse *(1 mark)*
BM *(1 mark)*
Urinalysis for glucose and ketones *(1 mark)*
Bloods – U+E, glucose *(1 mark)*
ABG *(1 mark)*

b *(1 mark for each correct answer, maximum 3 marks)* ___/3___
Insulin on sliding scale *(1 mark)*
Fluids *(1 mark)*
Potassium *(1 mark)*
Treatment of any underlying condition such as
infection *(1 mark)*

c Metabolic *(1 mark)* acidosis *(1 mark)* ___/2___

d Lack of insulin causes gluconeogenesis, lipolysis, ___/3___
and glycogenolysis *(1 mark)*, which all raise glucose
levels *(1 mark)* and produce ketones *(1 mark)*

Summary

Diabetic ketoacidosis carries a 5–10% morbidity, higher in the elderly. It often occurs in new type 1 diabetics, and in those diabetics
who gets an infection, causing loss of appetite, and they reduce their
insulin. It is caused by insulin deficiency, and hepatic overproduc-
tion of glucose and ketone bodies. The typical features are hyperglycaemia, which results in osmotic diuresis and dehydration. Raised
ketone levels causes metabolic acidosis, with a low bicarbonate,
under 12, indicating severe acidosis. Hyperkalaemia also occurs,
though overall potassium is depleted due to diuresis and vomiting.

8 a Acromegaly *(1 mark)* `/1`
  b Growth hormone *(1 mark)* `/2`
  Anterior pituitary *(1 mark)*
  c *(1 mark for each correct answer, maximum 3 marks)* `/3`
  Luteinising hormone *(1 mark)*
  Follicle stimulating hormone *(1 mark)*
  Thyroid stimulating hormone *(1 mark)*
  Adrenocorticotrophic hormone *(1 mark)*
  Prolactin *(1 mark)*
  d *(1 mark for each correct answer, maximum 4 marks)* `/4`
  Prognathism *(1 mark)*
  Thickening of skin *(1 mark)*
  Hoarseness *(1 mark)*
  Headache *(1 mark)*
  Sweating *(1 mark)*
  Weakness *(1 mark)*
  Joint pain *(1 mark)*
  Carpal tunnel syndrome *(1 mark)*
  Widely spaced teeth *(1 mark)*
  e *(1 mark for each correct answer, maximum 3 marks)* `/3`
  Hypertension *(1 mark)*
  Diabetes *(1 mark)*
  Hypopituitarism *(1 mark)*
  Cardiovascular disease *(1 mark)*
  Arthritis *(1 mark)*
  Visual abnormalities *(1 mark)*

Summary

Acromegaly is caused by a somatotroph adenoma of the anterior pituitary. Excess growth hormone can be diagnosed by high insulin-like growth factor 1 levels, or measuring growth hormone levels following an oral glucose tolerance test, as it should fall but will not fall in disease. CT or MRI can be used to locate the tumour. Surgery or bromocriptine can be used for treatment.

9 a *(maximum 2 marks)* `/2`
  SSRIs *(1 mark)* such as citalopram, fluoxetine,
    sertraline *(1 mark for any of these)*
  b Primary hyperparathyroidism *(1 mark)* `/1`
  c *(1 mark for each correct answer, maximum 3 marks)* `/3`
  Muscle weakness *(1 mark)*

Polyuria *(1 mark)*
Constipation *(1 mark)*
Kidney stones *(1 mark)*
Fatigue *(1 mark)*
Loss of appetite *(1 mark)*
Dehydration *(1 mark)*
Cardiac arrhythmias *(1 mark)*
Fractures *(1 mark)*
Pancreatitis *(1 mark)*
Coma *(1 mark)*

d *(1 mark for each correct answer, maximum 3 marks)* `/3`
Fluids *(1 mark)*
Diuretics *(1 mark)*
Bisphosphonates *(1 mark)*
Calcitonin *(1 mark)*

e Parathyroidectomy *(1 mark)* `/1`

f Promotes absorption of calcium from the gut `/3`
    (1 mark)
Increases osteoblast activity, thus promoting bone
    formation *(1 mark)*
Inhibits parathyroid hormone secretion *(1 mark)*

Summary

Primary hyperparathyroidism affects 0.1% of the population. It is commonly due to a single adenoma in one of the parathyroid glands, although it can occur due to hyperplasia or rarely carcinoma.

10 a *(1 mark for each correct answer, maximum 3 marks)* `/3`
Hyperthyroidism *(1 mark)*
Chronic renal failure *(1 mark)*
Renal artery stenosis *(1 mark)*
Phaechromocytoma *(1 mark)*
Cushing's *(1 mark)*
Acromegaly *(1 mark)*
Hyperparathyroidism *(1 mark)*

b Phaeochromocytoma *(1 mark)* `/1`

c Raised adrenaline increases the sympathetic `/3`
drive*(1 mark)* causing vasoconstriction *(1 mark)*
and tachycardia *(1 mark)*

d *(1 mark for each correct answer, maximum 3 marks)* `/3`
Pallor *(1 mark)*
Flushing *(1 mark)*

Sweating *(1 mark)*
Headache *(1 mark)*
Anxiety *(1 mark)*
Abdominal pain *(1 mark)*
Constipation *(1 mark)*
Weight loss *(1 mark)*

e Control hypertension and heart rate with the
use of alpha *(1 mark)* and beta blockers *(1 mark)*
in combination. `/2`

f Resection of the tumour *(1 mark)* `/1`

Summary

Phaechromocytomas are rare tumours which accounts for <0.1%
cases of hypertension. 10% are malignant, 10% are extra-adrenal,
10% are bilateral and 10% are familial, associated with neurofi-
bromatosis and multiple endocrine neoplasia type II (parathyroid
and pituitary tumours).

11 a *(1 mark for each correct answer, maximum 3 marks)* `/3`
Amenorrhoea *(1 mark)*
Loss of libido *(1 mark)*
Headache *(1 mark)*
Visual abnormalities *(1 mark)*

b Anterior *(1 mark)* pituitary *(1 mark)* `/2`

c Prolactin levels (>1000) *(1 mark)* `/2`
Cranial CT/MRI *(1 mark)*

d *(1 mark for each correct answer, maximum 2 marks)* `/2`
Medical (bromocriptine, pergoline, or cabergoline)
   (1 mark)
Radiotherapy *(1 mark)*
Surgical excision through a trans-sphenoidal
   approach *(1 mark)*

e Bitemporal hemianopia *(1 mark)* due to `/2`
compression of the optic chiasm *(1 mark)*

Summary

A prolactinoma is a tumour of the pituitary gland causing
excess secretion of prolactin. It commonly causes galactorrhoea,
amenorrhoea, hypogonadism and impotence, and if large may
cause headaches, visual field defects and hypopituitarism due to
compressive effects.

7 Rheumatology
QUESTIONS

1 Jean is 47. She presents to her GP complaining of widespread joint pains, stiffness and tiredness. After a number of tests you make a diagnosis of rheumatoid arthritis.
   a Give three tests you would order to make a
     diagnosis of RA.   *3 marks*
   b What two alternative diagnoses would you
     consider?   *2 marks*
   c Name four features of RA seen in the hands.   *4 marks*
   d Identify three types of medical therapy used
     to manage RA.   *3 marks*

2 Katie is 13. She loves horse riding and is a promising ballet dancer. One morning she wakes up and finds her knee swollen and is unable to move it. She cannot bear weight. Believing it to be a sports-related injury she tries simple 'RICE' therapy but after one week it is getting worse and she feels systemically unwell. Her mother brings her to see you, her GP.
   a Give three differential diagnoses.   *3 marks*
     The episode resolves with anti-inflammatories.
     However, one year later she re-presents with
     bilaterally swollen ankles and knees. She is unable
     to walk and her stepfather carries her into the GP
     surgery. Blood tests show Hb 9.0, CRP 236, ESR 43,
     WCC and neutrophils both normal.
   b What is the diagnosis?   *1 mark*
   c Give four features you would examine for apart
     from the joints.   *4 marks*
   d Explain what Felty's syndrome is.   *1 mark*
   e What advice would you give to Katie and her
     parents?   *2 marks*

Complete SAQs for Medical Finals By P. Stather et al, Published 2010 by Blackwell Publishing, ISBN: 978-1-4501-8928-6.

3 Maggie is 78. Her husband brings her to A & E as this morning Maggie was unable to move her left knee due to severe pain and she could not bear weight. Her husband thinks Maggie has broken her knee but cannot recollect her having any falls; x-ray of the joint reveals no fractures. Examination reveals temperature of 38.4°C, with a hot, swollen joint. You diagnose septic arthritis.

   a Give two other diagnoses you would consider.   *2 marks*

   b Apart from blood tests, what two further
investigations would you request?   *2 marks*

   c What organisms are commonly responsible for
septic arthritis in:

     i) infants?   *1 mark*

     ii) sexually active adults?   *1 mark*

   d Give three aspects of your management of
septic arthritis.   *3 marks*

   e Suggest two complications of this disease which
may ensue.   *2 marks*

   f Give two different ways infection may spread to
a joint.   *2 marks*

4 Mark is 46 years old. Although you are nominally listed as his GP you have never seen him in the five years he has lived in the area. He presents to you one Monday morning complaining of excruciating pain in his big toe which started on Saturday night.

   a How much alcohol does he drink daily/weekly?   *3 marks*

   b You note that Mark is overweight and after
weighing and measuring him estimate his BMI
to be 28. He also admits to drinking a bottle of red
wine a night with his partner. You suspect this to
be a case of acute gout. How could you prove
your diagnosis is correct?   *2 marks*

   c What two medications would you use to manage
Mark initially?   *2 marks*

   d Name two common side effects for each of the
above drugs   *2 marks*

   e Six months later Mark presents again, this time
with excruciating pain in his knee. He says it is
'exactly the same as before' and he can't bear for
the joint to be touched although after some
encouragement he allows you to aspirate the joint
and you make an appointment to see him again in

one month to discuss ways to prevent further
attacks. What long-term medication would you
now consider using to treat Mark and why would
you not use it in the acute phase?   *2 marks*
f   What two other methods could Mark employ to
decrease the risk of having another attack?   *2 marks*
g   If Mark's condition became chronic, suggest one
musculoskeletal feature you might see.   *1 mark*

5   Elizabeth is 68. She has cared for both of her elderly parents
until recently when her father passed away. She is still the main
carer for her mother who has moderate Alzheimer's disease. Her
one escape from her parents is working two days a week at a
charity shop but the other staff have recently been asking her to
take on more responsibility. She presents to her GP complaining
of headaches and scalp tenderness.
a   How much alcohol is she drinking daily/weekly?   *3 marks*
b   Give two differential diagnoses.   *2 marks*
c   Elizabeth also mentions that she gets pain in
her jaw when chewing her food. What two
further blood tests may be helpful to come
to a diagnosis?   *2 marks*
d   What other more invasive examination could be
performed to come to a definitive diagnosis and
what would be seen histologically?   *2 marks*
e   What is the diagnosis for Elizabeth?   *1 mark*
f   What is the most feared complication of this
condition?   *1 mark*
g   What medical treatment will you initiate, what
side-effects could it have and how will you prevent
the side-effect?   *2 marks*
h   Patients with this condition may also suffer from
polymyalgia rheumatica. Define this.   *1 mark*

6   Tom is 19 and in his first term at university. He limps into the
health centre complaining that his knee hurts and saying he
feels 'rough'. On examination you find he has a swollen knee
and a sausage-shaped toe as well as a high temperature. He says
that his knee has swollen in the past following an episode of
gastroenteritis.
a   What is the clinical term for a 'sausage-shaped toe'?   *1 mark*
b   Give two of your differential diagnoses.   *2 marks*

c As you have never met Tom you ask him if he has any other health problems. He coughs a bit and looks sheepish and after gentle persuasion admits he has some problems 'with his tackle'. What three questions would you ask to elicit the nature of these problems? *3 marks*

d What three investigations would you request? *3 marks*

e Bearing in mind Tom's revelation what is your final diagnosis? *1 mark*

f Give two aspects of your treatment of this condition. *2 marks*

g What is the name of the syndrome that encompasses arthritis, urethritis and conjunctivitis? *1 mark*

7 James is 37. He has been a patient at your surgery for 10 years and is known to have ankylosing spondylitis.

a What major histocompatibility complex antigen is associated with ankylosing spondylitis? *1 mark*

b Give three musculoskeletal features which may be seen in patients with ankylosing spondylitis. *3 marks*

c James is concerned because he has been researching his condition on the Internet and he sees that by his late 50s his posture, which is currently good, is likely to deteriorate. What is the name used to describe this posture? *1 mark*

d What test is used to assess flexion of the lumbar spine and how is it performed? *2 marks*

e Give three extraskeletal features which may be present in ankylosing spondylitis. *3 marks*

f On spinal x-ray of someone with ankylosing spondylitis, what will be seen? *1 mark*

8 Sarah is 43. She has suffered from Raynaud's phenomenon for 10 years. At an annual health check you notice that her appearance has changed.

a What is Raynaud's phenomenon? *1 mark*

b You believe Sarah may have developed limited cutaneous scleroderma (formerly known as CREST). Give three other features of this condition. *3 marks*

c Give three ways in which you would manage Sarah's Raynaud's. *3 marks*

d If you suspected diffuse cutaneous scleroderma, which organs would you investigate for involvement of the disease? **2 marks**

e How is the onset of diffuse cutaneous scleroderma different to limited cutaneous scleroderma? **1 mark**

9 Rebekah comes to the outpatients clinic. She has a diagnosis of systemic lupus erythematosus. Initially her condition was mild but repeated flares have caused long-term health problems and she now suffers significant arthralgia and arthritis which prevent her from working.

a Give three dermatological features which may be seen in SLE. **3 marks**

b Which five other systems may be affected by SLE? **5 marks**

c What serological abnormality is found in SLE? **1 mark**

d Give three medications which can be used to treat SLE. **3 marks**

10 Jeremy, a 25-year-old gentleman, presents to A & E with acute SOB and mild right-sided chest pain. On examination you are unable to hear breath sounds on the right side, and the x-ray reveals a pneumothorax. There has been no history of trauma, and he has not suffered from this in the past. He does not smoke; however, you notice that he is particularly tall.

a Describe two abnormalities you would see on chest x-ray of this gentleman. **2 marks**

b What is the immediate treatment of a spontaneous tension pneumothorax? **1 mark**

c You suspect Marfan's disease. Give three other signs and symptoms you would look for on examination. **3 marks**

d Give two other possible complications which may occur in the future. **2 marks**

e What is the genetic defect in Marfan's disease? **1 mark**

f Give one long-term treatment to prevent recurrent pneumothoraces. **1 mark**

Rheumatology

ANSWERS

1 a *(1 mark for each correct answer, maximum 3 marks)* `/3`
FBC – looking for anaemia of chronic disease,
thrombocytosis secondary to inflammation or
leucopenia of Felty's syndrome *(1 mark)*
ESR/CRP/plasma viscosity – raised in response to
presence of synovitis *(1 mark)*
Rheumatoid factor – present in the serum of 70–90%
of patients but is often not detectable during the
initial few months of the disease *(1 mark)*
Anti-CCP – a very specific test for RA which helps
predict the level of joint damage likely to occur
(1 mark)

b *(1 mark for each correct answer, maximum 2 marks)* `/2`
Septic arthritis *(1 mark)*
Reactive arthritis *(1 mark)*
Reiter's syndrome *(1 mark)*
Psoriatic arthritis *(1 mark)*

c *(1 mark for each correct answer, maximum 4 marks)* `/4`
Rheumatoid nodules *(1 mark)*
Ulnar deviation of fingers *(1 mark)*
Radial deviation of wrist *(1 mark)*
Synovitis of wrists *(1 mark)*
Synovitis of metacarpophalangeal joints *(1 mark)*
Synovitis of interphalangeal joints *(1 mark)*
Wasting of small muscles of the hand *(1 mark)*
Fixed deformity of the wrists and hands *(1 mark)*
Scars from previous operations *(1 mark)*
Boutonniere deformity *(1 mark)*
Swan neck deformity *(1 mark)*
Z deformity of thumb *(1 mark)*

d *(1 mark for each correct answer, maximum 3 marks)* `/3`
NSAIDs *(1 mark)*
Corticosteroids *(1 mark)*

DMARDs (disease-modifying anti-rheumatic drugs)
(1 mark)
Biological therapies *(1 mark)*

Summary

Rheumatoid arthritis is a chronic disabling condition that is characterised by a symmetrical polyarthritis. The cause of rheumatoid arthritis is unknown but there is an increased incidence in those patients who have a positive family history and there is also an association with HLA-DR4 in most ethnic groups. In RA the synovium is infiltrated by chronic inflammatory cells and then proliferates out over the surface of the cartilage to form a pannus.

2 a *(1 mark for each correct answer, maximum 3 marks)* `/3`
Septic arthritis *(1 mark)*
RA *(1 mark)*
Meniscal damage *(1 mark)*
Trauma *(1 mark)*
Ligamentous damage *(1 mark)*
Hamarthrosis *(1 mark)*

 b Juvenile rheumatoid arthritis *(1 mark)* `/1`

 c *(1 mark for each correct answer, maximum 4 marks)* `/4`
Anaemia *(1 mark)*
Anterior uveitis *(1 mark)*
Evanescent rash *(1 mark)*
Hepatomegaly *(1 mark)*
Splenomegaly *(1 mark)*
Lymphadenopathy *(1 mark)*

 d Association of RA with splenomegaly and leucopenia, `/1`
which usually happens in patients who are
rheumatoid factor positive *(1 mark)*

 e *(1 mark for each correct answer, maximum 2 marks)* `/2`
Continue with sporting activities as much as possible,
especially hydrotherapy *(1 mark)*
Physiotherapy *(1 mark)*
Many children with RA grow out of the condition
(1 mark)

Summary

There are a number of different subtypes of juvenile rheumatoid arthritis, all of which carry slightly different clinical features and prognosis. Generally speaking, however, juvenile RA is seen more commonly in girls than boys. It is important to acknowledge that whilst many children do grow out the disease (it burns itself out) others are left with a long-term disability or active arthritis into their adulthood.

3 a *(1 mark for each correct answer, maximum 2 marks)* `/2`
Osteomyelitis *(1 mark)*
Gout *(1 mark)*
Reactive arthritis *(1 mark)*
b Ultrasound of joint, looking for effusion *(1 mark)* `/2`
Aspiration of joint – sent for Gram stain, culture and
examination for crystals *(1 mark)*
c i) *Haemophilus influenzae (1 mark)* `/2`
ii) *Neisseria gonorrhoeae (1 mark)*
d *(1 mark for each correct answer, maximum 3 marks)* `/3`
Analgesia *(1 mark)*
Splinting *(1 mark)*
Antibiotics *(1 mark)*
Surgical drainage and washout *(1 mark)*
e *(1 mark for each correct answer, maximum 2 marks)* `/2`
Seeding of infection can occur to other organs
(1 mark)
Recurrence of infection *(1 mark)*
Joint destruction with long-term arthritis or
ankylosis *(1 mark)*
Avascular necrosis *(1 mark)*
f *(1 mark for each correct answer, maximum 2 marks)* `/2`
Spread via haematogenous route *(1 mark)*
Direct spread from metaphysis *(1 mark)*
Penetrating trauma/surgery *(1 mark)*

Summary
Septic arthritis occurs after a joint is infected with a pyogenic organism such as *Staphylococcus aureus*. Patients present with an extremely painful, red, swollen joint, and are unable to bear weight. It is a medical emergency and treatment (as above) will ensure the minimal possible damage to the joint.

4 a *(1 mark for each correct answer, maximum 3 marks)* `/3`
Has he ever had anything like this previously?
(1 mark)

Can he bear weight or move the joint? *(1 mark)*

Any history of trauma? *(1 mark)*

Is the toe painful to touch? *(1 mark)*

Does he have any other medical problems currently? *(1 mark)*

Does he take any medications (including over-the-counter preparations)? *(1 mark)*

How much alcohol does he drink daily/weekly? *(1 mark)*

What type of foods does he regularly include in his diet (e.g. shellfish)? *(1 mark)*

Has he recently been on a diet, and how much does he weigh? *(1 mark)*

b *(1 mark for each correct answer, maximum 2 marks)* `/2`

Blood tests – hyperuricaemia, raised CRP and ESR, polymorphonuclear leucocytosis *(1 mark)*

Random blood glucose (followed up as appropriate depending on results) *(1 mark)*

Needle aspiration of joint and synovial fluid analysis by microscopy (urate crystals are needle-shaped and birefringent) *(1 mark)*. Aspiration may be difficult in small joints.

X-ray – rule out any traumatic cause *(1 mark)*

c Colchicines *(1 mark)* `/2`

Corticosteroids if the patient can't tolerate NSAIDs or colchicines *(1 mark)*

d *(1 mark for each correct answer, maximum 2 marks)* `/2`

NSAIDs – GI upset, renal failure *(1 mark)*

Colchicine – diarrhoea, nausea, vomiting, abdominal pain, renal impairment, rash *(1 mark)*

Corticosteroids – GI upset, long-term osteoporosis *(1 mark)*

e Allopurinol *(1 mark)* – in the acute phase will precipitate an attack of gout *(1 mark)* `/2`

f Lose weight (slowly and sensibly on a balanced diet with regular exercise) *(1 mark)* `/2`

Reduce the amount of alcohol he consumes *(1 mark)*

g *(1 mark maximum)* `/1`

Gouty tophi *(1 mark)*

Joint deformity due to bony erosion and cartilage destruction *(1 mark)*

Summary

Gout occurs when there is an abnormality of uric acid metabolism which leads to the deposition of urate acid crystals within the joint. The crystals are ingested by neutrophils which initiates a pro-inflammatory reaction that is characterised by severe pain that is exquisitely sensitive to touch, and swollen joints. Patients with gout often complain that they feel even the touch of a sheet is too painful to bear.

5 a *(1 mark for each correct answer, maximum 3 marks)* /3
   What type of pain is it? *(1 mark)*
   Is the pain increased by coughing, sneezing, etc?
      (1 mark)
   Any flashing lights, visual disturbance? *(1 mark)*
   Any feelings of nausea? *(1 mark)*
   Has she noticed any change in her mood? *(1 mark)*
   Any weight loss? *(1 mark)*
   Any change in sleeping habits? *(1 mark)*
   What medication is she taking? *(1 mark)*
   Is she drinking 2 litres of water a day? *(1 mark)*
   How much alcohol is she drinking daily/weekly? *(1 mark)*
   Any history of neck problems? *(1 mark)*

 b *(1 mark for each correct answer, maximum 2 marks)* /2
   SLE *(1 mark)*
   Temporal/giant cell arteritis *(1 mark)*
   Polyarteritis nodosa *(1 mark)*
   Tension headache *(1 mark)*

 c *(1 mark for each correct answer, maximum 2 marks)* /2
   ESR – greatly elevated, 60–100 mm h^{-1} (although
      very rarely may be normal) *(1 mark)*
   CRP – raised *(1 mark)*
   Plasma alpha2 globulins – raised *(1 mark)*
   Albumin – occasionally reduced *(1 mark)*
   FBC – normochromic, normocytic anaemia
      (1 mark)

 d Superficial temporal artery biopsy /2
   (1 mark) – characteristic granulomatous changes
   within arterial wall, such as lymphocytes, plasma
   cells, multinucleate cells, and destruction of internal
   elastic lamina *(1 mark)*. The disease is patchy so
   excise over 1 cm.

 e Temporal/giant cell arteritis *(1 mark)* /1

f Blindness due to ischaemic optic neuritis *(1 mark)* /1

g High dose steroids *(1 mark)* – risk of osteoporosis /2
so need to prescribe bisphophonate *(1 mark)*

h Weakness of proximal muscles which may also /1
be tender *(1 mark)*. Patients present with
symmetrical pain and stiffness in the shoulder
and pelvic girdles, and a peripheral synovitis
affecting medium-sized joints is common.

Summary

Temporal/giant cell arteritis typically affects the elderly. It is often seen in conjunction with polymyalgia rheumatica. The most feared complication is blindness, but if the temporal arteritis affects the vertebrobasilar or carotid circulations the patient may suffer a stroke.

6 a Dactylitis *(1 mark)* /1

b *(1 mark for each correct answer, maximum 2 marks)* /2
Rheumatoid arthritis *(1 mark)*
Septic arthritis *(1 mark)*
Osteomyelitis *(1 mark)*
Reactive arthritis *(1 mark)*
Reiter's syndrome *(1 mark)*

c *(1 mark for each correct answer, maximum 3 marks)* /3
Any urinary symptoms? *(1 mark)*
Is he sexually active? *(1 mark)*
How many partners has he had? *(1 mark)*
Does he always use barrier protection during
intercourse? *(1 mark)*
Did he have the urogenital problems before his knee
and toe began to trouble him? *(1 mark)*

d *(1 mark for each correct answer, maximum 3 marks)* /3
FBC *(1 mark)*
CRP/ESR *(1 mark)*
Urethral swabs *(1 mark)*
Urine microscopy, culture and sensitivity *(1 mark)*

e Reactive arthritis *(1 mark)* /1

f *(1 mark for each correct answer, maximum 2 marks)* /2
NSAIDs *(1 mark)*
Local corticosteroids – once septic arthritis has been
ruled out *(1 mark)*

Disease-modifying anti-rheumatic drugs *(1 mark)*
Antibiotics if an organism can be isolated *(1 mark)*
Referral to GUM *(1 mark)*

g Reiter's syndrome *(1 mark)* /1

Summary

Reactive arthritis is seen most commonly in males. It is a seron-egative synovitis triggered by a recent infection. The precipitating infection is usually of a gastrointestinal or genitourinary origin. In patients for whom the infection is of a GU origin it is important that contact tracing (which can be done anonymously by the local GUM clinic) is carried out.

7 a HLA B27 *(1 mark)* /1
   b *(1 mark for each correct answer, maximum 3 marks)* /3
     Lower back pain *(1 mark)*
     Stiffness – worse early in morning and after long
       periods of rest *(1 mark)*
     Stiffness improves with exercise *(1 mark)*
     Postural deformity *(1 mark)*
     Reduction of chest expansion *(1 mark)*
     Tenderness of sacroiliac joints *(1 mark)*
     Reduced mobility of lumbar spine *(1 mark)*
   c Question mark posture *(1 mark)* /1
   d Schober test *(1 mark)* – a pen mark is made on /2
     the skin at the lumbosacral joint at the level
     of the dimples of Venus. A second mark is
     placed 10 cm above. On bending forward with
     straight legs the marks should separate by 5 cm.
     (1 mark)
   e *(1 mark for each correct answer, maximum 3 marks)* /3
     Anorexia *(1 mark)*
     Fatigue *(1 mark)*
     Weight loss *(1 mark)*
     Fever *(1 mark)*
     Acute anterior uveitis *(1 mark)*
     Ascending aortitis *(1 mark)*
     Aortic incompetence *(1 mark)*
     Cardiac dysrhythmias *(1 mark)*
     Pulmonary fibrosis *(1 mark)*
     Amyloidosis *(1 mark)*

f Bamboo spine appearance – due to squaring $\boxed{/1}$
of vertebrae, formation of syndesmophytes
and ossification of longitudinal ligaments
(1 mark)

Summary

Ankylosing spondylitis is associated with the HLA B27 antigen. Typical presentation is of a young man (in his 20s) who suffers increasing pain and morning stiffness in the lower back. Loss of lumbar lordosis and an increased kyphosis results in the typical 'question mark' posture.

8 a Spasm of the arteries supplying the fingers $\boxed{/1}$
and toes, which is associated with cold
(1 mark)
b *(1 mark for each correct answer, maximum 3 marks)* $\boxed{/3}$
Calcinosis *(1 mark)*
Oesophagitis *(1 mark)*
Sclerodactyly *(1 mark)*
Telangiectasia *(1 mark)*
c *(1 mark for each correct answer, maximum 3 marks)* $\boxed{/3}$
Hand warmers *(1 mark)*
Battery-powered gloves *(1 mark)*
Oral vasodilators – calcium channel blockers, ACE
inhibitors *(1 mark)*
Sympathectomy *(1 mark)*
d *(1 mark for each correct answer, maximum 2 marks)* $\boxed{/2}$
Renal system *(1 mark)*
Respiratory system *(1 mark)*
Cardiovascular system *(1 mark)*
e Limited usually starts with Raynaud's, whereas $\boxed{/1}$
diffuse begins with oedema before skin sclerosis
follows *(1 mark)*

Summary

Systemic sclerosis is a multisystem disease which can have widespread clinical features. It carries the poorest prognosis of all the scleroderma-related conditions. There is no known cause for systemic sclerosis but there are a number of environmental risk factors for developing scleroderma-like disorders, such as exposure to silica dust or vinyl chloride.

9 a *(1 mark for each correct answer, maximum 3 marks)* /3
  Photosensitivity *(1 mark)*
  'Butterfly rash' over the nose and cheeks *(1 mark)*
  Discoid lupus – demarcated, pigmented or
    atrophic plaques *(1 mark)*
  Hair loss/alopecia *(1 mark)*
  Mucosal ulceration of nose, mouth, vagina
    (1 mark)
  Cutaneous vasculitis *(1 mark)*

b *(1 mark for each correct answer, maximum 5 marks)* /5
  Cardiovascular *(1 mark)*
  Respiratory *(1 mark)*
  Renal *(1 mark)*
  Neurological *(1 mark)*
  Haematological *(1 mark)*
  Gastrointestinal *(1 mark)*

c *(maximum 1 mark)* /1
  Raised levels of double-stranded DNA *(1 mark)*
  Low C3 and C4 complement levels *(1 mark)*

d *(1 mark for each correct answer, maximum 3 marks)* /3
  NSAIDs *(1 mark)*
  Hydroxychloroquine *(1 mark)*
  Corticosteroids *(1 mark)*
  Steroid-sparing drugs such as azathioprine and
    methotrexate *(1 mark)*
  Cyclophosphamide *(1 mark)*

Summary

Systemic lupus erythematosus is a multisystem inflammatory disorder. Whilst the skin changes and arthralgia are the clinical features seen most commonly, the most life-threatening complications are those which affect the kidneys and brain. Although SLE is found in all ethnic groups it has the greatest prevalence amongst African American women. In SLE there is widespread vasculitis affecting all vessels and deposits of fibrinoid are found in both the blood vessels and tissues.

10 a *(1 mark for each correct answer, maximum 2 marks)* /2
  Loss of lung markings on the right *(1 mark)*
  Mediastinal shift *(1 mark)*
  Raised hemidiaphragm *(1 mark)*

b Needle aspiration *(1 mark)* /1

c *(1 mark for each correct answer, maximum 3 marks)* /3
Arachnodactyly *(1 mark)*
Wide arm span *(1 mark)*
High arched palate *(1 mark)*
Lens dislocation *(1 mark)*
Pectus excavatum/carinatum *(1 mark)*
Scoliosis *(1 mark)*
Flat feet *(1 mark)*
Micrognathia *(1 mark)*
Hypotonia *(1 mark)*
Hypermobile joints *(1 mark)*

d *(1 mark for each correct answer, maximum 2 marks)* /2
Aortic regurgitation *(1 mark)*
Bacterial endocarditis *(1 mark)*
Aortic aneurysm *(1 mark)*
Heart failure *(1 mark)*
Mitral valve prolapse *(1 mark)*
Visual problems *(1 mark)*
Scoliosis *(1 mark)*

e Defect in fibrillin-1 gene *(1 mark)* /1

f Pleurodesis *(1 mark)* /1

Summary

Marfan's syndrome is an autosomal dominant genetic condition that affects the connective tissues of all of the body's organs. The criteria for diagnosis states that two out of three major body organs must be affected before a diagnosis is made; otherwise an incorrect diagnosis could have disastrous consequences for an individual ranging from medical and psychological problems, to difficulty finding work and financial problems (e.g. getting a mortgage). Worldwide approximately 1 in 5000 people are affected and are at risk of dying from cardiovascular complications such as aortic aneurysm.

8 Elderly Medicine and Palliative Care

QUESTIONS

1 Betty is 84. Her relatives found her trying to cook her tea in the washing machine. She did not appear to recognise them and kept asking where her mother was. She has been admitted to the medical admissions unit with a mental state examination score of 3/30.

   a Give four additional questions you would ask in the history. **4 marks**

   b FBC, U+E, CRP, LFT, haematinics, calcium, magnesium, phosphate, TFTs and glucose were sent. Suggest four other investigations you would request and what abnormalities might you see? **4 marks**

   c You treat Betty with a short course of empirical antibiotics and her condition improves. Her MMSE score improves to 28/30, thus confirming that this was an acute confusional state. Define delirium and explain how it differs from dementia. **2 marks**

   d Give three different categories of the MMSE. **3 marks**

2 Robert is admitted via 999. He was found on the floor by his carer. It is possible that he was on the floor for up to 10 hours. He had been incontinent of urine and faeces. It is unclear whether he lost consciousness. There is no other collateral history and Robert is unable to give a history as he is so upset and shaken.

   a Identify five possible causes for his collapse. **5 marks**

   b Give two measures you could take to prevent Robert from collapsing again. **2 marks**

   c Suggest three other members of the multidisciplinary team who may be able to offer positive help for Robert's care. **3 marks**

Complete SAQs for Medical Finals By P. Stather et al, Published 2010 by Blackwell Publishing, ISBN: 978-1-4501-8928-6.

3 Joan is 88. She lives with her disabled husband and is his main carer. They have meals on wheels but receive no other outside help and have no family. Joan is admitted to A & E having collapsed. Her husband reports she has recently been complaining of feeling dizzy and has been unsteady on her feet whenever she stands up. Joan has a past medical history of hypertension and angina. After examining her you diagnose postural hypotension.

a What is considered a significant postural drop?   *1 mark*

b Name three different classes of medications she may be taking for the above conditions, which can cause postural hypotension.   *3 marks*

c Taking a holistic viewpoint, give three ways in which you will proceed to look after Joan.   *3 marks*

d What medication could you start to prevent further postural drops?   *1 mark*

e When she feels better, Joan also reveals that she has been taking her GTN spray with increased frequency. By what mechanism does GTN work?   *1 mark*

f Name two of the common side-effects of nitrates.   *2 marks*

4 You have been Catharine's GP for 12 years. Two years ago she was diagnosed with advanced breast cancer and has recently been told she has widespread metastases in her liver and bones and that her condition is now considered terminal. She comes to your GP surgery requesting something to help her sleep at night.

a Suggest two things that might be causing Catharine's sleeplessness.   *2 marks*

b Name one medication which could be used to help her sleep.   *1 mark*

c Describe the analgesic ladder.   *3 marks*

d Give two other ways in which you could approach pain management in this patient.   *2 marks*

e Suggest two other means of support you can offer Catharine and her family.   *2 marks*

f If Catharine becomes unable to swallow, how else could you deliver medications? Name four.   *4 marks*

5 Tony is 58. He attends your GP surgery with his wife. She does most of the talking and he appears to be withdrawn. Tony's wife reports that he has become increasingly forgetful and recently she had a phone call from his work saying he hadn't turned up. He was found later that day wandering around the town centre asking people how to get home. He scores 15 out of 30 in his MMSE. After a few visits a diagnosis of dementia is made.

a Give three of the more common types of dementia. **3 marks**

b Name one medication he may be started on and how does it work? **2 marks**

c Suggest five sources of support Tony and his wife may be able to get help from. **5 marks**

6 Margaret is 64. She is brought to A & E by her husband because her speech has become slurred and she has a facial droop. Her symptoms resolve within 12 hours of admission, leaving no residual weakness. You make a diagnosis of TIA.

a Identify five risk factors for suffering a TIA or stroke. **5 marks**

b Give four tests you would consider arranging. **4 marks**

c Name two medications you would consider starting Margaret on. **2 marks**

d Suggest three lifestyle modifications you would encourage. **3 marks**

7 John is 78. He tried to phone his son in the early hours of the morning but was incomprehensible. The son went to his father's house and found his father collapsed on the floor. A maximum duration of 45 minutes had passed before John was taken to hospital. The next day on examination you find John has significantly decreased power in his left arm and leg, and weakness in the left side of his face. His reflexes were decreased and left sided plantars were upgoing. John has not recovered his speech and is unable to swallow.

a What is the likely diagnosis? **1 mark**

b What types of stroke are there? **2 marks**

c Where is the likely occlusion? **1 mark**

d Which two healthcare professionals can assess swallowing? **2 marks**

e Suggest three steps you can take to ensure John has a good outcome. **3 marks**

f How soon after a stroke would you try to reduce John's blood pressure? **1 mark**

8 Jane is 73. She comes to your GP surgery very upset because she has 'had a few accidents lately'. On further questioning she reveals she has involuntarily passed urine a number of times although in between these incidents she retains control of her bladder.

a Suggest five further questions you would ask her. **5 marks**

b Give two investigations you would perform. **2 marks**

c Name three methods you could use to help Jane. **3 marks**

9 You are working as a GP and are asked to go and see Mavis who is 87 and lives in a nursing home for people who suffer from dementia. Mavis's dementia means she is unable to communicate verbally with staff but they know her well and report that she is distressed by an itchy rash of 4 days' duration. After examining her you make a diagnosis of scabies.

a Give two characteristics of the rash that is associated with scabies. *2 marks*

b Give two sites in particular which you would examine if you suspected a diagnosis of scabies in any patient. *2 marks*

c What medication would you prescribe to treat the scabies? *1 mark*

d What advice would you give to the nursing home regarding their other residents and staff? *1 mark*

e Another well-known infestation is with lice. What is the medical name for head lice? *1 mark*

f How do head lice spread? *1 mark*

g How may head lice present? *2 marks*

10 Hortense is a 78-year-old lady of African origin. Her family bring her to A & E because she has been complaining of severe facial pain which she describes as similar to an electric shock and lasting only a few seconds. This has been occurring repeatedly for nearly a week, leading you to suspect Hortense has trigeminal neuralgia.

a Give four specific triggers for this pain which you would ask any patient about. *4 marks*

b What class of drug might you prescribe for the treatment of trigeminal neuralgia? *1 mark*

c Other than idiopathic, give two causes of trigeminal neuralgia. *2 marks*

d Name the three divisions of the trigeminal nerve. *1 mark*

e If Hortense had informed you she had recently had chicken pox or shingles your differential diagnosis would have included post-herpetic neuralgia. Give one risk factor known to increase the likelihood of developing this condition. *1 mark*

f Which drug may prove beneficial for patients with post-herpetic neuralgia? *1 mark*

Elderly Medicine and Palliative Care

ANSWERS

1 a *(1 mark for each correct answer, maximum 4 marks)*   /4
Pre-morbid functioning *(1 mark)*
Past medical history *(1 mark)*
Medications *(1 mark)*
Social circumstances *(1 mark)*
Any past similar episodes *(1 mark)*

b *(1 mark for each correct answer, maximum 4 marks)*   /4
Urine dipstick and MSU – infection markers,
   i.e. blood, protein, leukocytes, nitrites
   (1 mark)
CT head – presence of global atrophy, infarcts or
   space-occupying lesion *(1 mark)*
Blood culture – identify micro-organisms *(1 mark)*
Nursing observations – high temperature,
   tachycardia *(1 mark)*
CXR – focus of consolidation *(1 mark)*
AXR – constipation or obstruction *(1 mark)*

c Delirium is an acute confusional state with   /2
   fluctuating level of consciousness *(1 mark)*
Dementia is a global decline in cognition and has a
   progressive course with no changes in the level of
   consciousness *(1 mark)*

d *(1 mark for each correct answer, maximum 3 marks)*   /3
Orientation *(1 mark)*
Registration *(1 mark)*
Attention and calculation *(1 mark)*
Recall *(1 mark)*
Language *(1 mark)*

Summary

Delirium is an acute confusional state associated with a fluctuating level of consciousness. There are many causes which should be considered but one of the most common causes of a delirious state in a previously well individual is infection, which can be investigated very easily.

2 a *(1 mark for each correct answer, maximum 5 marks)*   **/5**
    Infection *(1 mark)*
    Seizure *(1 mark)*
    TIA *(1 mark)*
    Stroke *(1 mark)*
    Postural hypotension *(1 mark)*
    MI *(1 mark)*
    Dehydration *(1 mark)*
    Mechanical fall *(1 mark)*
    Hypoglycaemia *(1 mark)*
    Vestibular hypofunction *(1 mark)*

 b *(1 mark for each correct answer, maximum 2 marks)*   **/2**
    Reassess the need for antihypertensive medication
       (1 mark)
    OT home assessment to check for causes of
       mechanical fall *(1 mark)*
    Appropriate medication to prevent stroke/TIA
       (1 mark)

 c *(1 mark for each correct answer, maximum 3 marks)*   **/3**
    OT – to provide any necessary aids and equipment
       (1 mark)
    Physiotherapist – to improve mobility *(1 mark)*
    Rehabilitation hospital – build confidence prior to
       discharge *(1 mark)*
    ENT opinion – Looking for vestibular causes *(1 mark)*
    Optician – to ensure there are no cataracts or the
       need for glasses *(1 mark)*
    Dietician – so an adequate diet can be made to avoid
       dehydration and malnutrition *(1 mark)*
    Referral to the falls clinic *(1 mark)*

Summary

Falls are a very common cause for hospital admission in the elderly, and the cause is often not found. It is however important to screen for the above conditions and involve the multidisciplinary team in the care of these patients to ensure that further falls are prevented, as next time it might lead to fractures, head injuries or other problems.

3 a A decrease in systolic blood pressure of over
20 mmHg on standing up *(1 mark)* | /1 |

b *(1 mark for each correct answer, maximum 3 marks)* | /3 |
Diuretics *(1 mark)*
ACE inhibitors *(1 mark)*
Nitrates *(1 mark)*
Beta-blockers *(1 mark)*
Alpha-blockers *(1 mark)*

c *(1 mark for each correct answer, maximum 3 marks)* | /3 |
Alter medications *(1 mark)*
OT referral *(1 mark)*
Falls prevention class *(1 mark)*
Ensure there is appropriate care for her husband
   (1 mark)
Increased help at home *(1 mark)*
Physiotherapy *(1 mark)*

d Fludrocortisone *(1 mark)* | /1 |

e Decreases preload on the heart by vasodilating all | /1 |
blood vessels, but predominantly the veins (1 mark)

f *(1 mark for each correct answer, maximum 2 marks)* | /2 |
Headache *(1 mark)*
Dizziness *(1 mark)*
Nausea and vomiting *(1 mark)*
Postural drop *(1 mark)*
Tachycardia *(1 mark)*
Flushing *(1 mark)*
Heartburn *(1 mark)*
Rash *(1 mark)*

Summary
Postural hypotension should be measured by taking the blood pressure while the patient is lying down, then letting the patient stand for 2 minutes and taking the blood pressure again. Postural hypotension commonly occurs due to polypharmacy or incorrect or overuse of antihypertensives by patients. Dizziness and falls are the most common symptoms. Postural hypotension may be treated by stopping antihypertensives or with steroids if not iatrogenic.

4 a *(maximum 2 marks)* | /2 |
Physical pain *(1 mark)*
Anxiety *(1 mark)*

Depression *(1 mark)*

b *(maximum 1 mark)*   /1

Zopiclone *(1 mark)*

Temazepam or other benzodiazepine *(1 mark)*

c Simple analgesia (paracetamol or NSAIDs which   /3
    work particularly well with bone pain) *(1 mark)*

Weak opiates (codeine) *(1 mark)*

Strong opiates (morphine) *(1 mark)*

It is important to prescribe regular pain relief
    rather than wait for the pain to come on, with
    alternative analgesia for breakthrough pain.

d *(1 mark for each correct answer, maximum 2 marks)*   /2

Palliative radiotherapy *(1 mark)*

Emotional/psychological/spiritual support *(1 mark)*

TENS machine *(1 mark)*

e *(1 mark for each correct answer, maximum 2 marks)*   /2

Involvement of Macmillan/palliative care team *(1 mark)*

CBT *(1 mark)*

Hospice care *(1 mark)*

f *(1 mark for each correct answer, maximum 4 marks)*   /4

IM *(1 mark)*

IV *(1 mark)*

S/C *(1 mark)*

S/L *(1 mark)*

Topical *(1 mark)*

PEG *(1 mark)*

Summary

Terminal care is a difficult subject for many healthcare professionals. It is important to appreciate that there may be many different
causes for pain and suffering amongst terminal patients and their
families. The best way to ascertain what each individual needs is
to make sure you allow them plenty of time to talk openly in a
supportive environment.

5 a *(1 mark for each correct answer, maximum 3 marks)*   /3

Alzheimer's disease *(1 mark)*

Vascular dementia *(1 mark)*

Lewy body *(1 mark)*

Wernicke's encephalopathy *(1 mark)*

Fronto-temporal dementia *(1 mark)*

b *(maximum 2 marks)* /2
Donepezil – acetylcholinesterase inhibitor increases
levels of acetylcholine in the brain *(2 marks)*
Memantine – NMDA receptor antagonist which
increases glutamate transmission in the brain
(2 marks)

c *(1 mark for each correct answer, maximum 5 marks)* /5
Alzheimer's Society *(1 mark)*
GP *(1 mark)*
Local support groups such as Age Concern *(1 mark)*
OT *(1 mark)*
Physiotherapy *(1 mark)*
Day hospitals *(1 mark)*
Respite care *(1 mark)*

Summary

The incidence of dementia increases with age. 1% of those under
65 are affected, whereas 6% of 75–79-year-olds are affected, and
45% of those over 95. The uncommon causes are Pick's disease,
Huntington's chorea, Parkinson's disease, CJD, hypothyroidism,
diabetes, anoxia, space-occupying lesions, and head trauma or
infection.

6 a *(1 mark for each correct answer, maximum 5 marks)* /5
Hypertension *(1 mark)*
Diabetes *(1 mark)*
Increasing age *(1 mark)*
Hypercholesterolaemia *(1 mark)*
Heart valve abnormalities *(1 mark)*
Abnormal heart rhythms *(1 mark)*
Family history *(1 mark)*
Past medical history – previous stroke/TIA
(1 mark)
Presence of circulating antibodies (e.g. lupus)
(1 mark)
OCP *(1 mark)*
Alcohol *(1 mark)*
Smoking *(1 mark)*

b *(1 mark for each correct answer, maximum 4 marks)* /4
Fasting lipid profile *(1 mark)*
FBC (for platelets) *(1 mark)*

U+Es (renal disease may cause hypertension)
(1 mark)
USS carotids *(1 mark)*
ECG *(1 mark)*
Echocardiogram *(1 mark)*
Circulating antibody profile (ANCA, ANA) *(1 mark)*
CT head *(1 mark)*
c *(1 mark for each correct answer, maximum 2 marks)* `/2`
Aspirin *(1 mark)*
Statin *(1 mark)*
Antihypertensives at a later stage *(1 mark)*
d *(1 mark for each correct answer, maximum 3 marks)* `/3`
Healthier diet *(1 mark)*
Stop smoking *(1 mark)*
Stop drinking alcohol *(1 mark)*
Increase exercise *(1 mark)*

Summary

Having a TIA or recurrent TIAs is a risk factor for suffering a more serious stroke in the future. It is therefore important to investigate patients with TIAs so that any abnormalities can be managed appropriately to reduce the risk of suffering a major stroke. TIAs are commonly caused by AF and carotid stenosis and treatment of the underlying cause may prevent further more serious events in the future.

7 a CVA *(1 mark)* `/1`
  b Ischaemic *(1 mark)* `/2`
    Haemorrhagic *(1 mark)*
  c Posterior circulation *(1 mark)* `/1`
  d Nurse (with special training) *(1 mark)* `/2`
    SALT *(1 mark)*
  e *(1 mark for each correct answer, maximum 3 marks)* `/3`
    Refer to specialist stroke unit *(1 mark)*
    Consider NG tube/PEG *(1 mark)*
    Begin secondary prevention strategies, such as
      aspirin (unless it's haemorhagic), a statin, and
      antihypertensives *(1 mark)*
    Early physiotherapy and occupational therapy
      (1 mark)
  f After the first 2 weeks *(1 mark)* `/1`

Summary

The posterior circulation is supplied by the basilar artery. The common signs and symptoms of stroke are diplopia, bilateral visual loss, dysarthria, dysphagia, unsteadiness, amnesia and unilateral weakness with contralateral facial weakness. Basilar artery occlusion is frequently fatal.

8 a *(1 mark for each correct answer, maximum 5 marks)* `/5`
Any recent UTI symptoms? *(1 mark)*
Does this happen on coughing/sneezing/laughing?
(1 mark)
Does this happen because she doesn't realize she
needs to pass urine? *(1 mark)*
Does this happen because she cannot get to the toilet
fast enough (i.e. problems with mobility)? *(1 mark)*
What medications does she take? *(1 mark)*
Does she drink lots of tea/coffee/cola? *(1 mark)*
Has she ever had abdominal surgery/hysterectomy?
(1 mark)
Has she ever had children? Were they difficult births
and heavy babies? *(1 mark)*
Does she have any strange sensations (e.g. like a
lump)? *(1 mark)*

b Urine dipstick and MC+S *(1 mark)* `/2`
Flow cystometry *(1 mark)*

c *(1 mark for each correct answer, maximum 3 marks)* `/3`
Advise pelvic floor exercises *(1 mark)*
Suggest products (such as pads) to help disguise
problem *(1 mark)*
Refer to urology or gynaecology consultant for
further investigation/surgery *(1 mark)*
Avoid caffeine *(1 mark)*
Ensure she isn't taking diuretics unnecessarily
(1 mark)
Consider starting medications such as oxybutynin if
neurogenic bladder is thought to be a factor *(1 mark)*

Summary

The psychological and social impact should not be overlooked. Regardless of age, incontinence is an embarrassing and socially isolating condition that has a substantial impact on patients' lives.

If the cause is found to be gynaecological, one of two procedures can be performed if the patient is suitable: a high vaginal tape or a colposuspension.

9 a *(1 mark for each correct answer, maximum 2 marks)* `/2`
Itchy red papules *(1 mark)*
Linear or curved skin burrows *(1 mark)*
Itching is worse at night *(1 mark)*

b *(1 mark for each correct answer, maximum 2 marks)* `/2`
Web spaces between fingers and toes *(1 mark)*
Palms of hands *(1 mark)*
Soles of feet *(1 mark)*
Around the wrists *(1 mark)*
Around the umbilicus *(1 mark)*
Around the nipples *(1 mark)*
Axillae *(1 mark)*
Male genitalia *(1 mark)*

c *(maximum 1 mark)* `/1`
Topical malathion *(1 mark)*
Topical 5% permethrin *(1 mark)*

d *(maximum 1 mark)* `/1`
All close contacts should be treated at the same time *(1 mark)*
Treat all skin below the neck in anybody over 2 years old *(1 mark)*

e Pediculosis capitis *(1 mark)* `/1`
f Direct contact *(1 mark)* `/1`
g *(1 mark for each correct answer, maximum 2 marks)* `/2`
Itchy scalp *(1 mark)*
Excoriations on scalp *(1 mark)*
Occasionally erythematous papules on neck *(1 mark)*
Presence of eggs bound tightly to hair shaft *(1 mark)*
In severe infestations adult lice may be seen *(1 mark)*

Summary

Infestations often invoke horror in people as they think of 'creepy crawlies'. It is important to educate people about simple measures they can take to prevent transmission. Examples of this would include patients with scabies having their own towels and bed linen that are washed separately from those of non-infected patients. As a GP you could see many parents who are upset that their child has head lice as they believe it is an indication of poor hygiene in the home. It is worth informing them that children easily pass head lice around at school and that it is no reflection on their own standards. They should be encouraged to use regular surveillance techniques such as wet combing with a detector comb and to treat according to local advice. Simple measures such as putting long hair into a ponytail may also be helpful.

10 a *(1 mark for each correct answer, maximum 4 marks)* ☐ **/4**
   Washing *(1 mark)*
   Shaving *(1 mark)*
   Touching a specific area *(1 mark)*
   Brushing teeth *(1 mark)*
   Brushing hair *(1 mark)*
   Cold wind *(1 mark)*
   Eating *(1 mark)*
 b *(maximum 1 mark)* ☐ **/1**
   Anticonvulsant, e.g. gabapentin *(1 mark)*
   Tricyclic antidepressant, e.g. amitriptyline *(1 mark)*
 c *(1 mark for each correct answer, maximum 2 marks)* ☐ **/2**
   Multiple sclerosis *(1 mark)*
   Lesions of the cerebellopontine angle *(1 mark)*
   Atrioventricular malformation *(1 mark)*
   Tumours of the fifth nerve, such as
     neuroma *(1 mark)*
 d Ophthalmic, maxillary, mandibular *(1 mark)* ☐ **/1**
 e *(maximum 1 mark)* ☐ **/1**
   Age *(1 mark)*
   Late treatment with acyclovir *(1 mark)*
 f Amitriptyline *(1 mark)* ☐ **/1**

Summary

Trigeminal neuralgia is also known as tic douloureux because of the characteristic way patients will screw their faces up during an attack. It is typically unilateral and is seen most commonly in older people. In a younger person with bilateral symptoms it is important to consider MS as an underlying cause. Post-herpetic neuralgia is also a condition that affects the elderly more frequently. It most commonly affects the ophthalmic division but it can occur anywhere.

9 Haematology

QUESTIONS

1 Philippe has rheumatoid arthritis which is reasonably well controlled on methotrexate. His GP regularly checks his bloods.

  a Explain which blood test is particularly important to check and why, when a patient is on methotrexate. *2 marks*

  b The GP also sends an FBC request. This shows a normocytic anaemia. Give three causes of a normocytic, normochromic anaemia. *3 marks*

  c Suggest two factors which affect the normal values for haemoglobin. *2 marks*

  d Give two signs associated with anaemia. *2 marks*

  e Give two symptoms a patient may present with other than tiredness. *2 marks*

2 Julie is 24. She presents to her GP complaining of feeling 'constantly exhausted'. Thyroid function tests are normal but FBC reveals a microcytic anaemia.

  a Give three further questions you would ask to elicit the possible cause of her microcytosis. *3 marks*

  b What further investigations would you request? Give three. *3 marks*

  c Other than pallor of the mucous membranes, give three other signs which may be present on examination of a patient with iron deficiency anaemia. *3 marks*

  d You decide to start ferrous sulphate TDS. Give two side-effects Julie may experience. *2 marks*

3 Thomas is 48. He presents to his GP complaining of feeling tired all the time. After examining him the GP notes a number

Complete SAQs for Medical Finals By P. Stather et al, Published 2010 by Blackwell Publishing, ISBN: 978-1-4501-8928-6.

of signs suggestive of anaemia and requests an FBC which is reported as being consistent with a macrocytosis.

a Other than vitamin B12 or folate deficiency, give three causes of a macrocytosis. *3 marks*

b Vitamin B12 deficiency may be caused in a number of different ways. State three ways and give an example for each. *6 marks*

c Where is vitamin B12 primarily absorbed? *1 mark*

d What type of gait is seen in patients with severe long-term vitamin B12 deficiency? *1 mark*

e What is necessary for the absorption of vitamin B12? What is its deficiency called? And how would you test for this condition? *3 marks*

4 Matthew is 45. He is referred to haematology outpatients by his GP who had done some recent blood tests, the results of which are consistent with an acute leukaemia.

a What four general features are seen in a patient with acute leukaemia? *4 marks*

b Bone marrow failure will lead to which three abnormalities being seen on routine haematology? *3 marks*

c Give two causes of acute myeloid leukaemia other than 'de novo'. *2 marks*

d Both AML and ALL may have specific characteristics not seen in the other. Suggest what they are. *2 marks*

5 Malcolm is 74. He approached his GP complaining of a palpable lump in the left side of his abdomen. The GP is concerned about the possibility of chronic lymphocytic leukaemia and has referred to you for a second opinion. On examination you find evidence of hepatic enlargement, splenic enlargement and generalized painless lymphadenopathy.

a Give two features which distinguish the spleen from other organs on examination. *2 marks*

b Bearing in mind the physical findings, you too suspect a possible diagnosis of chronic lymphocytic leukaemia (CLL). What three other symptoms will you ask about? *3 marks*

c What staging system is used to stage CLL? *1 mark*

d Give one way that CML is different to CLL in its progression. *1 mark*

e Malcolm does not handle news of his diagnosis well; he becomes increasingly withdrawn and often mentions that he has considered suicide rather than 'waiting for the inevitable'. Who could you consider referring Malcolm to in order to offer him the support he requires? Give three suggestions. *3 marks*

6 Gregory is 78. He has recently been given a diagnosis of non-Hodgkin's lymphoma (NHL).

a Other than idiopathic give four risk factors for developing NHL. *4 marks*

b What are the two types of NHL seen on lymph node histology? *2 marks*

c If the disease spreads what symptoms may he complain of? Suggest four. *4 marks*

7 Alan is 27. After extensive investigation for a number of non-specific complaints a diagnosis of Hodgkin's lymphoma is made.

a Name the system used to stage Hodgkin's and explain the different stages. *1+4 marks*

b What investigation would you use to diagnose Hodgkin's and what would you expect to see? *2 marks*

c Which virus is associated with Hodgkin's lymphoma? *1 mark*

d Give four symptoms which a patient with Hodgkin's may complain of. *4 marks*

8 You are on duty in A & E when an ambulance brings in a 23-year-old male of Afro-Caribbean descent who is screaming and writhing in pain. It turns out Jamal is well known to your department as he suffers from sickle cell disease.

a How is sickle cell disease inherited genetically? *1 mark*

b Jamal says his sickle cell was diagnosed after a sickle test. What three features may be seen on routine haematology and a blood film to support this diagnosis? *3 marks*

c This crisis turns out to be due to a bone crisis. Give two ways of managing Jamal. *2 marks*

d Patients with sickle cell are known to suffer from acute chest syndrome. Give three features of acute chest syndrome. *3 marks*

e Explain why you might give prophylactic penicillin
to adult sickle cell patients. *1 mark*

f If Jamal were to have a child with his current
partner (who has been tested for sickle cell and is
not a carrier) what is the percentage chance that
they may have i) a child without sickle cell or trait
ii) a child with sickle trait iii) a child with sickle
cell disease? *1 mark*

9 Demetrius is referred to paediatric out patients by his GP. He is
6 months old and appears malnourished. On taking a detailed
history you find out that Demetrius' mum and dad are both
originally from Greece and that Demetrius has failed to thrive
since birth but recently he has seemed more floppy and lethargic. Blood tests show anaemia and an MCV of 68fL.

a What type of anaemia is this? *1 mark*

b You suspect that Demetrius may suffer from
ß-thalassaemia major. Why is it unlikely that
he suffers from α-thalassaemia major? *1 mark*

c Give four clinical features you would examine
for if you suspected a diagnosis of beta-thalassaemia
major. *4 marks*

d Give one feature seen on a laboratory blood film
in this condition. *1 mark*

e What treatment would you initiate in order to
facilitate normal development? *1 mark*

f Give one long-term complication of the above
treatment and explain how you would prevent
this occurring. *2 marks*

g If Demetrius developed hypersplenism and
needed a splenectomy, what vaccine would he
be given and why? *2 marks*

10 Max is 68. You have been his GP for some years and are aware
that he has MGUS (monoclonal gammopathy of unknown sig-
nificance). His wife brings him to an appointment one day saying he is constantly tired and weak.

a What is MGUS? *1 mark*

b Explain what myeloma is. *1 mark*

c Explain why the kidneys are commonly affected
in myeloma. *2 marks*

d Give three investigations used to diagnose
myeloma and explain what abnormality you
would see in each. *3 marks*

e Give two mechanisms which could explain the
development of anaemia in patients with
myeloma. *2 marks*

f Explain why patients may suffer from bone pains
and hypercalcaemia. *2 marks*

g Give three causes for confusion in a patient with
myeloma. *3 marks*

11 Elizabeth is 58. She is referred to the anticoagulation clinic
prior to surgery to fit an artificial heart valve. The valve will
not be a Starr-Edwards valve. She will require anticoagulation
with warfarin.

a What will be the target INR you aim for? *1 mark*

b What is the mechanism by which warfarin acts? *1 mark*

c How would you initiate the warfarin
postoperatively? *1 mark*

d Elizabeth does well after surgery until five
days postoperatively when she has a nose bleed.
You phone the lab to request her INR to be done
as an urgent and the INR is subsequently reported
as 9.7. Give three steps you will take. *3 marks*

e Give three drugs/classes of drugs which exhibit
antiplatelet activity thus decreasing the risk of
clot formation. *3 marks*

f There are many drugs which interact with
warfarin. Name one drug which decreases the
activity of warfarin and one drug which
potentiates the effects of warfarin. *2 marks*

12 John is 20 months. His mum and dad bring him to hospital for the fourth time in six months. In a similar presentation to the previous episodes they say his knee has swollen
and they can give no explanation for how it occurred. An
x-ray reveals no damage to the bones and the longer that
John is kept in the department the more distressed his father
becomes. He keeps shaking his head and saying he knew
they shouldn't come to A & E, he bruises easily too and
when he was young his parents were accused of abusing him
because of all the bruises. At this the consultant paediatrician

starts asking more questions about his father's bruising and suggests that both John and his dad should have blood tests to investigate the possibility they may both have a problem with their blood clotting. These tests reveal they both have haemophilia A.

a Other than haemophilia, name another
common inherited disorder of coagulation.   *1 mark*

b How is haemophilia inherited genetically?   *1 mark*

c What clotting factor is implicated in
haemophilia A?   *1 mark*

d John's haemophilia is described as severe whilst
his dad's is only mild. What clues do you have
from the history to support this?   *2 marks*

e Give one medical and one social way of managing
John's condition.   *2 marks*

f If you were concerned about the possibility of a
non-accidental injury in any child, give two
important steps you would take.   *2 marks*

g Disseminated intravascular coagulation is an
acquired clotting disorder. What is the pathological
basis for this condition?   *2 marks*

Haematology

ANSWERS

1 a *(1 mark for each correct answer, maximum 2 marks)* $\boxed{/2}$
Liver function tests (AST and albumin)
(1 mark) – methotrexate is metabolized by the
liver thus it can disturb liver function *(1 mark)*
FBC *(1 mark)* – methotrexate may cause bone
marrow suppression *(1 mark)*

b *(1 mark for each correct answer, maximum 3 marks)* $\boxed{/3}$
Chronic infections, e.g. TB, osteomyelitis *(1 mark)*
Inflammatory diseases, e.g. RA, connective tissue
disorders *(1 mark)*
Malignant disease *(1 mark)*
Endocrine disorders (e.g. hypothyroidism,
hypopituitarism, hypoadrenalism) *(1 mark)*
Renal failure *(1 mark)*
Acute blood loss *(1 mark)*
Haemolysis *(1 mark)*
Bone marrow hypoplasia *(1 mark)*
Pregnancy *(1 mark)*

c *(1 mark for each correct answer, maximum 2 marks)* $\boxed{/2}$
Age *(1 mark)*
Race *(1 mark)*
Sex *(1 mark)*
Altitude *(1 mark)*

d *(1 mark for each correct answer, maximum 2 marks)* $\boxed{/2}$
Pallor (palm of hands, mucous membranes) *(1 mark)*
Koilonychia (spoon shaped nails) *(1 mark)*
Tachycardia *(1 mark)*
Tachypnoea *(1 mark)*
Systolic flow murmur *(1 mark)*

e *(1 mark for each correct answer, maximum 2 marks)* $\boxed{/2}$
Breathlessness *(1 mark)*
Headaches *(1 mark)*
Faintness *(1 mark)*

Intermittent claudication *(1 mark)*

Peripheral oedema *(1 mark)*

Palpitations *(1 mark)*

Angina (if underlying coronary artery disease, the presence of anaemia may exacerbate symptoms) *(1 mark)*

Summary

Anaemia of chronic disease may be associated with either a microcytic or normocytic anaemia. Normocytic, normochromic anaemia is also seen following an acute blood loss (e.g. significant GI bleed). However, it is worth remembering that after a large bleed, although the patient's blood pressure will drop, their haemoglobin will remain steady initially until the dilutional effects of the fluid replacement have taken place.

2 a *(1 mark for each correct answer, maximum 3 marks)* `/3`

Does she suffer from heavy periods? *(1 mark)*

Is she pregnant? *(1 mark)*

Any weight loss? *(1 mark)*

Any change in bowel habit? (inflammatory bowel disease or coeliac disease) *(1 mark)*

Is she following a diet which limits her food intake? *(1 mark)*

Has she recently noticed she has lost any blood when she goes to the toilet? *(1 mark)*

Is she vegetarian? *(1 mark)*

Has she suffered from any nose bleeds recently? *(1 mark)*

Is she aware of any blood conditions that run in her family? *(1 mark)*

Any exposure to lead? *(1 mark)*

b *(1 mark for each correct answer, maximum 3 marks)* `/3`

Blood film *(1 mark)*

Serum iron and iron binding capacity *(1 mark)*

Serum ferritin *(1 mark)*

Serum soluble transferring receptor *(1 mark)*

Bone marrow aspirate *(1 mark)*

Coeliac antibodies *(1 mark)*

c *(1 mark for each correct answer, maximum 3 marks)* `/3`

Brittle nails *(1 mark)*

Atrophy of the papillae of the tongue (smooth tongue) *(1 mark)*

Angular stomatitis *(1 mark)*
Brittle hair *(1 mark)*
Koilonychia (spoon-shaped nails) *(1 mark)*
d *(1 mark for each correct answer, maximum 2 marks)* $\boxed{/2}$
Nausea *(1 mark)*
Constipation or diarrhoea *(1 mark)*
Epigastric pain *(1 mark)*
Black stool *(1 mark)*

Summary

Young women who may be vegetarian or suffer from heavy menstrual loss commonly present complaining of feeling tired and lethargic leading to a diagnosis of iron deficiency anaemia. Microcytic anaemia may be caused by iron deficiency, thalassaemia, sideroblastic anaemia, lead poisoning or chronic disease. It is important to educate patients on the importance of a well balanced diet as well as warning them of the potential side effects of the medication you prescribe. Iron salts (especially modified release preparations) may cause diarrhoea when taken in some patients whilst others may experience constipation and pass black stools.

3 a *(1 mark for each correct answer, maximum 3 marks)* $\boxed{/3}$
Alcohol (*1 mark*)
Liver disease *(1 mark)*
Hypothyroidism *(1 mark)*
Pregnancy *(1 mark)*
Reticulocytosis *(1 mark)*
b *(1 mark for each correct answer, maximum 6 marks)* $\boxed{/6}$
Reduced intake *(1 mark)* – vegans *(1 mark)*
Reduced absorption in the stomach
    (1 mark) – gastrectomy *(1 mark)*
Reduced absorption in the small intestine
    (1 mark) – Crohn's disease, ulcerative colitis, ileal
    resection, ileal TB *(1 mark)*
Increased utilization *(1 mark)* – blind loop syndrome
    (bacterial overgrowth) or fish tapeworm *(1 mark)*
Abnormal metabolism *(1 mark)* – transcobalamin II
    deficiency *(1 mark)*
Drugs *(1 mark)* – nitrous oxide, metformin *(1 mark)*
c Terminal ileum *(1 mark)* $\boxed{/1}$
d High stepping gait *(1 mark)* $\boxed{/1}$

e Intrinsic factor *(1 mark)*   /3
Pernicious anaemia *(1 mark)*
Schilling test or anti-parietal cell antibody *(1 mark)*

Summary

Macrocytic red blood cells have an MCV exceeding 95 fL. The condition may be attributed to folate deficiency, vitamin B12 deficiency or megaloblastic anaemia. If due to dietary deficiency, treatment is by dietary supplementation. If a patient's haemoglobin drops significantly or if they are asymptomatic, they can be transfused.

4 a *(1 mark for each correct answer, maximum 4 marks)*   /4
Breathless *(1 mark)*
Feverish *(1 mark)*
Pale *(1 mark)*
Minor splenic enlargement *(1 mark)*
Minor lyphadenopathy *(1 mark)*
Purpura *(1 mark)*
Bleeding gums *(1 mark)*
Fatigue *(1 mark)*
b Anaemia *(1 mark)*   /3
Neutropenia *(1 mark)*
Thrombocytopenia *(1 mark)*
c *(1 mark for each correct answer, maximum 2 marks)*   /2
Other haematological malignancy – CML *(1 mark)*,
    paroxysmal nocturnal haemoglobinuria *(1 mark)*,
    polycythaemia rubra vera *(1 mark)*
Previous exposure to radiation – workplace or as medical treatment *(1 mark)*
Previous chemotherapy *(1 mark)*
d AML – Auer rods seen in 30% *(1 mark)*   /2
ALL – Philadelphia chromosome *(1 mark)*

Summary

Leukaemia is a malignancy of the bone marrow and is broadly subdivided into acute and chronic. Acute leukaemia has a much faster course than chronic leukaemia and without treatment may be fatal within a few weeks. ALL is most commonly seen in young children (where it carries a good prognosis) whilst AML is seen more commonly with increasing age and carries a poorer prognosis.

5 a *(1 mark for each correct answer, maximum 2 marks)*   /2
Notched edge *(1 mark)*

Moves with respiration *(1 mark)*
Can't palpate above it *(1 mark)*
b *(1 mark for each correct answer, maximum 3 marks)*   /3
Fever *(1 mark)*
Weight loss *(1 mark)*
Night sweats *(1 mark)*
Recurrent infections *(1 mark)*
Symptoms of anaemia (tiredness, lethargy, etc.)
    (1 mark)
c ABC *(1 mark)*   /1
d In CML there may be myeloid transformation after   /1
2–5 years and give rise to an acute leukaemia
(either AML or ALL) *(1 mark)*
e *(1 mark for each correct answer, maximum 3 marks)*   /3
Palliative care *(1 mark)*
Macmillan cancer support *(1 mark)*
GP *(1 mark)*
Psychotherapist *(1 mark)*
Local cancer/leukaemia support groups for patients
    and families affected by the disease *(1 mark)*

Summary

Chronic leukaemia is subdivided into chronic lymphocytic and chronic myeloid leukaemia. CML presents in middle age with lethargy, weight loss, night sweats and left upper quadrant pain. CLL is the most common leukaemia in the world and may be asymptomatic. CLL symptoms can include malaise, weight loss, night sweats, bleeding and recurrent infections.

6 a *(1 mark for each correct answer, maximum 4 marks)*   /4
HIV *(1 mark)*
Drugs such as cyclosporin A, steroids, chemotherapy
    (1 mark)
Radiation for treatment of Hodgkin's lymphoma or
    other malignancies *(1 mark)*
Rheumatoid arthritis *(1 mark)*
Systemic lupus erythematosus *(1 mark)*
Sjogren's disease *(1 mark)*
Herbicides *(1 mark)*
Wiskott-Aldrich syndrome *(1 mark)*
Ataxia telangiectasia *(1 mark)*

b High grade – such as diffuse large B cell, Burkitt ⬚ /2
     lymphoma, and anaplastic large cell
     lymphoma *(1 mark)*
    Low grade – such as follicular lymphoma, mantle
     cell, small cell lymphocytic, or MALT lymphoma
     (1 mark)
c *(1 mark for each correct answer, maximum 4 marks)* ⬚ /4
    Fever *(1 mark)*
    Weight loss *(1 mark)*
    Anaemia *(1 mark)*
    Bleeding *(1 mark)*
    Night sweats *(1 mark)*
    Infection *(1 mark)*
    Lymph node masses *(1 mark)*
    Extranodal masses *(1 mark)*

Summary

Grading of lymphoma is dependant on the speed of growth of the cancerous cells, with low-grade lymphoma being slow growing and less aggressive than the rapidly dividing high-grade lymphomas. Low-grade lymphomas may change into a more aggressive high-grade lymphoma over time in 15–30% of patients, and some patients may have features of both low- and high-grade lymphoma at the same time.

7 a Ann Arbor system *(1 mark)* ⬚ /5
    I-a single nodular region or a single extra
     nodular site
    II-Two or more nodal regions or an extra nodal site
     and regional nodal involvement on the same
     side of the diaphragm
    III-Lymphatic enlargement on both sides of the
     diaphragm
    IV-Liver or bone marrow involvement or significant
     involvement of another extra lymphatic site
    (½ mark each, 4 marks if all correct)
b Lymph node biopsy *(1 mark)* ⬚ /2
    Reed-Sternberg cells *(1 mark)*
c Epstein Barr virus *(1 mark)* ⬚ /1
d *(1 mark for each correct answer, maximum*
    4 marks) ⬚ /4

Palpable lumps *(1 mark)*
Fever *(1 mark)*
Weight loss *(1 mark)*
Malaise *(1 mark)*
Pruritus *(1 mark)*
Superior vena caval obstruction *(1 mark)*
Lymph node pain on ingestion of alcohol *(1 mark)*

Summary

Patients with lymphoma may present with lymph node enlargement, fever, drenching night sweats and weight loss. On examination you may also detect hepatosplenogemaly, as well as concurrent signs of anaemia. Treatment is dependent upon stage of disease and may include chemotherapy and radiotherapy.

8 a Autosomal recessive *(1 mark)*   `/1`
  b Sickle shaped cells *(1 mark)*   `/3`
    Features of splenic atrophy (Howell-Jolly bodies
      present in red blood cells) *(1 mark)*
    Moderate anaemia of between 7 and 9 g/dL
      (1 mark)
  c *(1 mark for each correct answer, maximum 2 marks)*   `/2`
    Analgesia using simple analgesics or opiate-based
      ones *(1 mark)*
    High fluid intake (either orally or intravenously)
      (1 mark)
    Oxygen therapy *(1 mark)*
    Antibiotics *(1 mark)*
    Folic acid *(1 mark)*
  d *(1 mark for each correct answer, maximum 3 marks)*   `/3`
    Rapid onset of chest pain *(1 mark)*
    Rapid progression of chest pain *(1 mark)*
    Hypoxia *(1 mark)*
    Cough *(1 mark)*
    Bilateral lung infiltrates *(1 mark)*
  e Patients may suffer from hyposplenism and thus   `/1`
    require prophylaxis against encapsulated
    bacteria *(1 mark)*
  f i) 0% *(1/3 mark)*
    ii) 100% *(1/3 mark)*
    iii) 0% *(1/3 mark)*   `/1`

Summary

As Jamal suffers from sickle cell disease he must have two sickle cell chromosomes, one of which must be passed on to any of his children. His partner has no sickle cell chromosomes, so every child will be a carrier only, except in exceptionally rare new genetic mutations, or gene transcription errors. Patients with sickle cell will require genetic counselling to explain to them the risks of offspring being affected.

9 a Microcytic *(1 mark)* `/1`

b α-thalassaemia major (otherwise known as `/1`
hydrops fetalis) often ends in intrauterine
death. He would have been unlikely to
survive gestation. *(1 mark)*

c *(1 mark for each correct answer, maximum 4 marks)* `/4`
Frontal bossing of skull *(1 mark)*
Hepatomegaly *(1 mark)*
Splenomegaly *(1 mark)*
Signs of recurrent infections (e.g. fever) *(1 mark)*
Leg ulcers *(1 mark)*
Jaundice *(1 mark)*
General body habitus (looking for signs of wasting)
(1 mark)

d *(maximum 1 mark)* `/1`
Target cells *(1 mark)*
Nucleated red cells *(1 mark)*

e Blood transfusion *(1 mark)* `/1`

f Iron overload *(1 mark)* `/2`
Chelation with desferrioxamine *(1 mark)*

g Pneumovax *(1 mark)* – to protect against `/2`
encapsulated organisms *(1 mark)*
You should also ensure that Hib and meningitis C
vaccines have been given previously.

Summary

Not all patients with thalassaemia have thalassaemia major. Thalassaemia trait (which may be alpha or beta) occurs when there is one normal and one abnormal globin gene. In both alpha and beta traits there is a mild anaemia. Partners of people who carry thalassaemia trait should be tested prior to beginning a family as if they too carry the trait there is a risk their offspring could have thalassaemia major. The disease is more common in Mediterranean countries and countries where malaria is endemic as it offers protection against malaria. In countries where the prevalence of thalassaemia is high, genetic testing and counselling before couples get married is routine.

10 a A monoclonal paraprotein without other features of myeloma *(1 mark)* `/1`

b In myeloma there is a clone of cancerous plasma cells which fill the bone marrow and produce only a single immunoglobulin type (an M band). *(1 mark)* `/1`

c *(1 mark for each correct answer, maximum 2 marks)* `/2`
Normally plasma cells produce an equal ratio of heavy:light chains but in myeloma the regulation of this process is disrupted and an excess of light chains is produced (Bence Jones proteins) *(1 mark)*. Bence Jones proteins are deposited in the kidney thus interfering with its function *(1 mark)*
Renal function is also affected by dehydration, drugs, infection and hypercalcaemia *(1 mark)*

d *(1 mark for each correct answer, maximum 3 marks)* `/3`
Serum electrophoresis – monoclonal immunoglobulin *(1 mark)*
Skeletal survey – lytic lesions in long bones, spine and skull. Skull has a typical 'pepper pot' appearance *(1 mark)*
Bone marrow examination – excess plasma cells *(1 mark)*
FBC – low Hb *(1 mark)*
U+E – high creatinine *(1 mark)*
LFT – low albumin in chronic disease *(1 mark)*
Urine collection for Bence Jones protein *(1 mark)*

e *(1 mark for each correct answer, maximum 2 marks)* `/2`
Tumour infiltration *(1 mark)*
Renal impairment *(1 mark)*
Cytokine mediated anaemia of chronic disease *(1 mark)*

f Myeloma cells release cytokines which stimulate osteoclast cells to erode bone leading to bone pains, lytic lesions and fractures *(1 mark)* as well as hypercalcaemia due to the excess calcium `/2`

released from the bone into the bloodstream.
(1 mark)

g Hyperviscosity syndrome *(1 mark)* `/3`
Hypercalcaemia *(1 mark)*
Infection *(1 mark)*

Summary

Myeloma is more common in the black community. The abnormal immunoglobulin production causes suppression of the production of normal immunoglobulin thus increasing susceptibility to infection. Patients may experience confusion due to hyperviscosity syndrome, hypercalcaemia or sepsis.

11 a 2.0–3.0 *(1 mark)* `/1`
  b Warfarin is a vitamin K antagonist which `/1`
    inhibits the carboxylation of clotting factors
    (1 mark)
  c Take baseline INR and then commence an IV `/1`
    heparin infusion and warfarin concurrently
    until the INR reaches a therapeutic level and
    is maintained at such for two consecutive
    days. *(1 mark)*
  d *(1 mark for each correct answer, maximum 3 marks)* `/3`
    Manage the nose bleed – if minor manage on ward
      with simple measures (i.e. ice, pressure). If nose
      bleed significant – contact ENT to consider packing
      (1 mark)
    Give vitamin K according to local protocol
      (1 mark)
    Seek advice from anticoagulation team/
      haematologist on call *(1 mark)*
    Withhold warfarin until INR is lower *(1 mark)*
  e *(1 mark for each correct answer, maximum 3 marks)* `/3`
    Aspirin *(1 mark)*
    Clopidogrel *(1 mark)*
    Dipyridamole *(1 mark)*
    Platelet IIb/IIIa receptor inhibitors (e.g. abciximab)
      (1 mark)
  f Drugs which decrease activity – antibiotics, `/2`
      laxative, cimetidine, phenylbutazone *(1 mark)*
    Drugs which increase activity – aspirin, antiplatelet
      drugs, alcohol *(1 mark)*

Summary

Warfarin efficacy is measured using INR which is a calculation of the patient's prothrombin time divided by the mean normal prothrombin time. Patients are advised to carry a card with them at all times which states that they are on warfarin in case they are ever taken to hospital in an emergency.

12 a *(maximum 1 mark)* /1

Von Willebrand's disease *(1 mark)*

Factor V Leiden *(1 mark)*

Antiphospholipid syndrome *(1 mark)*

b X-linked recessive *(1 mark)* /1

c Factor VIII *(1 mark)* /1

d Dad's is only mild because it only affects /2
him as 'bruising easily', he does not suffer spontaneous bleeding into his joints and he has not been diagnosed until adulthood (common in mild cases). *(1 mark)*

John's is severe because he suffers spontaneous bleeding into his joints and it has been identified in infancy/childhood. *(1 mark)*

e Medical – Regular prophylactic treatment /2
with factor VIII, parents to have training to be able to give further treatment if John has an accident in the home. *(1 mark)*

Social – advise to avoid rough play/contact sports. Ensure home is accident proofed. *(1 mark)*

f *(1 mark for each correct answer, maximum 2 marks)* /2
Explain your concerns to a senior doctor. *(1 mark)*

Document injuries with photographs if appropriate. *(1 mark)*

Contact the child protection liaison nurse/on call social worker for child protection. *(1 mark)*

g An insult (such as septicaemia or an obstetric /2
emergency) triggers the activation of the clotting cascade resulting in systemic microvascular thrombosis *(1 mark)*. The high consumption of coagulation factors can lead to bleeding but it is usually the end organ damage (e.g. renal damage) that leads to the high mortality rate *(1 mark)*

Summary

Haemophilia A and B are indistinguishable clinically but the difference occurs where B is caused by a deficiency of factor IX. Haemophilia A affects approximately 1 in 5000 males and is divided according to the amount of factor VIII present (mild >5%, moderate <5%, <1% severe). The most common inherited bleeding disorder is von-Willebrand's disease which may be mildly present in up to 1% of the population. The vWF may be either deficient or defective thus preventing clots from forming correctly. Patients with vWF present with skin bleeding, recurrent epistaxis and menorrhagia. Treatment is with desmopressin (if mild as this raises levels of circulating vWF) or with factor VIII concentrate if severe.

10 Infectious Diseases

QUESTIONS

1 Anthony, a 35-year-old, has recently returned from a business trip to Thailand. He presents with a 2-day history of urethral discharge and pain on passing urine. On examination he has a purulent urethral discharge from his penis.

   a Outline five aspects of a sexual history.   *5 marks*

   b What three investigations will you carry out?   *3 marks*

   c A Gram stain shows the presence of
      Gram-negative diplococci. What is the diagnosis?   *1 mark*

   d Which antibiotic will you prescribe for him?   *1 mark*

   e Suggest two pieces of advice you would give him.   *2 marks*

2 Olive, a 19-year-old girl who is sexually active, presents to you with some vaginal discharge and a fever. She has had multiple sexual partners and often forgets to use contraception.

   a Other than *Chlamydia*, give four infective causes
      of vaginal discharge.   *4 marks*

   b Give three tests which are available for the
      detection of *Chlamydia*.   *3 marks*

   c Name two complications of untreated *Chlamydia*. *2 marks*

   d What antibiotic will you prescribe to treat it?   *1 mark*

   e How do men present with *Chlamydia*?   *1 mark*

   f Olive's forgetfulness also exposes her to the
      possibility of pregnancy which she does not want.
      Give three different contraceptive methods she
      could use which may be suitable for her.   *3 marks*

3 Billy, a 31-year-old male, presents to you feeling very worried as whilst having a shower he noticed a painless ulcer on the tip of his penis. He last had unprotected sex around 3 weeks ago.

Complete SAQs for Medical Finals By P. Stather et al, Published 2010 by Blackwell Publishing, ISBN: 978-1-4501-8928-6.

On examination a painless chancre lesion is present and he has some painless inguinal lymphadenopathy.

a What is the likely diagnosis and causative organism? *2 marks*

b Give two ways in which the organism can be transmitted. *2 marks*

c What two tests would you request? *2 marks*

d What antibiotic will you prescribe and for how long? *2 marks*

e Name three late complications of untreated syphilis. *3 marks*

f Give three symptoms of congenital syphilis in a young baby. *3 marks*

4 Jake, a 17-year-old sexually active male, presents to you with symptoms of headache, fever and groin pain for 12 days. On examining him you notice multiple painful ulcers resembling herpes simplex virus surrounding his penis with inguinal lymphadenopathy.

a Name two other causes of genital ulcers. *2 marks*

b Identify two locations where you may commonly find herpes simplex ulcers. *2 marks*

c Give two complications of this disease. *2 marks*

d How can recurrent attacks occur? *1 mark*

e Give three ways in which you can manage the condition. *3 marks*

f What advice will you give him? *3 marks*

5 Seth is a 49-year-old male intravenous drug abuser who immigrated to the UK from Haiti many years ago. He presents to you feeling generally unwell and on examination he is very cachectic, has oral candidiasis, generalised lymphadenopathy and splenomegaly. You suspect HIV.

a Give two blood test abnormalities which may be present. *2 marks*

b Briefly explain the pathology of the disease. *3 marks*

c Name three specific infections which are more commonly encountered in AIDS patients. *3 marks*

d Identify three classes of drugs used in the management of HIV. *3 marks*

e Give three ways the MDT approaches the care of patients with HIV. *3 marks*

6 Aaron, a 25-year-old male, has just got back from a 2-month stay in India. On returning he presents with a high fever of 4 days' duration and you suspect malaria.

   a What three signs or symptoms would you enquire about?   *3 marks*

   b Name one species responsible for this infection, and the transmitting vector   *2 marks*

   c Briefly explain how this infection is transmitted.   *2 marks*

   d Give two causes of anaemia relating to this condition.   *2 marks*

   e Name one complication of this disease.   *1 mark*

   f What investigation will you request to confirm the dignosis?   *1 mark*

   g Name one antimalarial medication.   *1 mark*

   h What two pieces of advice would you give to travellers visiting high-risk areas?   *2 marks*

7 Jimmy, a 13-year-old boy, is brought in to see you by his worried father. Jimmy has had a 3-day history of fever, headache, difficulty eating and today he has noticed bilateral jaw pain. On examination he has bilaterally enlarged parotid glands. On further questioning his father tells you that he has not been immunised with the MMR vaccine.

   a What is the likely diagnosis?   *1 mark*

   b Name the virus involved.   *1 mark*

   c Name three complications of this disease.   *3 marks*

   d Give two ways in which you will manage this condition.   *2 marks*

   e Name two contraindications to the MMR vaccine.   *2 marks*

   f Why is the incidence of this disease increasing?   *1 mark*

8 Mary, an 89-year-old nursing home resident, is seen by her GP because staff feel that she has become unwell and has a productive cough. Her GP assumed it was a chest infection and gave her a 10-day course of amoxicillin. This did not seem to help and he switched her to a broader-spectrum antibiotic, but she has now developed very foul-smelling diarrhoea, and stool cultures in hospital have grown *Clostridium difficile*.

   a Give three risk factors for developing *C. diff.*   *3 marks*

   b Name a major complication of this disease.   *1 mark*

   c Suggest four ways that *C. diff.* can be prevented and controlled in the hospital.   *4 marks*

   d Give three aspects of the management of *C. diff.*   *3 marks*

9 Nigel, a 79-year-old gentleman, is admitted to hospital from his nursing home as his venous leg ulcers have started oozing pus.

   a Give three signs you would look for on examination of venous ulcers. *3 marks*

   b You swab the ulcers, and cultures show that they are colonised by MRSA. Give three risk factors for contracting MRSA. *3 marks*

   c What three things can be done to prevent further spread of the infection around the ward? *3 marks*

   d What three sites are swabbed during routine MRSA screening? *3 marks*

10 You have recently started working in A & E when an urgent staff meeting is called. The head of department states that there has been an upsurge in the number of cases of influenza seen recently and he is concerned that this may be the start of an epidemic.

   a What is the difference between an epidemic and a pandemic? *2 marks*

   b Give two ways any infection may be transmitted. *2 marks*

   c What three coryzal symptoms may a patient with influenza present with? *3 marks*

   d Identify three groups of people who should be offered a yearly 'flu jab'. *3 marks*

Infectious Diseases

ANSWERS

1 a *(1 mark for each correct answer, maximum 5 marks)*　　　`/5`
Number of sexual contacts *(1 mark)*
Type of sex oral/genital/anal *(1 mark)*
Dates of intercourse *(1 mark)*
Partner's gender *(1 mark)*
Regular partner/casual partner/prostitutes
　(1 mark)
Contraception used *(1 mark)*
Previous STIs *(1 mark)*
Previous HIV tests *(1 mark)*

b *(1 mark for each correct answer, maximum 3 marks)*　　`/3`
Urethral swab/smears *(1 mark)*
Urine test *(1 mark)*
Rectal swabs and culture if indicated *(1 mark)*
Throat swabs if indicated *(1 mark)*
Blood for syphilis and HIV *(1 mark)*

c *Neisseria gonorrhoeae (1 mark)*　　`/1`
d Ciprofloxacin single dose (500 mg) *(1 mark)*　　`/1`
e *(1 mark for each correct answer, maximum 2 marks)*　　`/2`
Get all sexual contacts tested *(1 mark)*
Contact tracing *(1 mark)*
Contraception for the future *(1 mark)*

Summary

Neisseria gonorrhoeae is spread via sexual contact, with half of infected women being asymptomatic. Male symptoms include anterior urethritis which causes dysuria and discharge. When an STI is suspected it is important to screen for other infections as most are transmitted via the same route. Uptake of GU services is poor as many people are reluctant to go. Single-dose treatments and health promotion, family planning and contraceptive advice are highly beneficial.

2 a *(1 mark for each correct answer, maximum 4 marks)* `/4`
   Trachomatis *(1 mark)*
   Moniliasis *(1 mark)*
   Vaginal thrush *(1 mark)*
   Trichomonas vaginalis (1 mark)
   Bacterial vaginosis *(1 mark)*
   Genital herpes *(1 mark)*
   Tuberculosis *(1 mark)*

  b *(1 mark for each correct answer, maximum 3 marks)* `/3`
   Cell culture from swabs *(1 mark)*
   Direct fluorescent antibody (DIF) *(1 mark)*
   Enzyme immunoassay (EIA) *(1 mark)*
   Nucleic acid amplification test (NAAT) from urine
      (1 mark)

  c Infertility *(1 mark)* `/2`
   PID *(1 mark)*

  d Azithromycin stat dose or doxycycline for `/1`
   14 days *(1 mark)*

  e Men are usually asymptomatic *(1 mark)* `/1`

  f *(1 mark for each correct answer, maximum 3 marks)*
   Condoms *(1 mark)*
   Depot injection *(1 mark)*
   Coil *(1 mark)*
   Contraceptive implant *(1 mark)*
   Abstinence *(1 mark)*

Summary

Chlamydia trachomatis is very common but is asymptomatic in the majority of women, and if left untreated can lead to infertility. Symptoms can include vaginal discharge and lower abdominal pain and if the infection ascends then acute salpingitis can occur. Symptoms in men are those of urethral discharge and dysuria but over half are asymptomatic.

3 a Syphilis *(1 mark)* `/2`
   Treponema pallidum (1 mark)

  b Sexual contact *(1 mark)* `/2`
   Transplacentally (vertical transmission) *(1 mark)*

  c *(1 mark for each correct answer, maximum 2 marks)* `/2`
   Dark-ground microscopy *(1 mark)*
   Enzyme immuno assay (EIA) *(1 mark)*

Venereal Disease Research Laboratory test (VDRL)
  (1 mark)
Screen for other STIs *(1 mark)*
d Penicillin *(1 mark)* IM for at least 7 days *(1 mark)*   /2
e *(1 mark for each correct answer, maximum 3 marks)*   /3
  Aortic regurgitation *(1 mark)*
  Gumma lesions *(1 mark)*
  Neurosyphillis *(1 mark)*
  Death *(1 mark)*
  Tabes dorsalis *(1 mark)*
  Blindness *(1 mark)*
  Mental disorders *(1 mark)*
  Aneurysms *(1 mark)*
f Nasal discharge *(1 mark)*   /3
  Skin lesions *(1 mark)*
  Failure to thrive *(1 mark)*

Summary

Syphilis typically presents initially with a painless chancre lesion with secondary symptoms beginning 4–8 weeks later. Syphilis is being diagnosed with increasing frequency. When diagnosed early it is easily cured with a short course of antibiotics, but if untreated or treated too late irreversible tissue damages ensues which may result in permanent cardiac or neurological disability or even death.

4 a *(1 mark for each correct answer, maximum 2 marks)*   /2
  Molluscum contagiosum *(1 mark)*
  Syphilis *(1 mark)*
  Lymphogranuloma venereum *(1 mark)*
  Behcet's disease *(1 mark)*
  Scabies *(1 mark)*
  Balanitis *(1 mark)*
  Erythema multiforme *(1 mark)*
b *(1 mark for each correct answer, maximum 2 marks)*   /2
  Genital tract *(1 mark)*
  Rectum *(1 mark)*
  Mouth *(1 mark)*
c Aseptic encephalitis *(1 mark)*   /2
  Urinary retention *(1 mark)*
d By reactivaton of the virus which can lie   /1
  dormant in the dorsal root ganglion *(1 mark)*

e *(1 mark for each correct answer, maximum 3 marks)* /3

Bathe in warm water *(1 mark)*

Rest *(1 mark)*

Antivirals (aciclovir) *(1 mark)*

Analgesia *(1 mark)*

Cryotherapy *(1 mark)*

Topical preparations *(1 mark)*

f Warn about recurrent attacks *(1 mark)* /3

Avoid intercourse during time of infection *(1 mark)*

Condoms not always effective at preventing transmission of this virus because ulcers may be present on the perineum, however they will prevent transmission of other STIs so should still be used! *(1 mark)*

Summary

Herpes simplex virus is the commonest sexually transmitted infection worldwide with the highest incidence among the 16–25-year age group. Patients present with multiple painful ulcers around the genital region. Recurrent attacks are common as the virus is able to lie dormant and this can be managed well with simple measures such as bathing in warm water. Women with active HSV should avoid vaginal delivery as they risk vertical transmission to the baby.

5 a *(1 mark for each correct answer, maximum 2 marks)* /2

Lymphopenia *(1 mark)*

Thrombocytopenia *(1 mark)*

Low CD4 count *(1 mark)*

Reversed CD4:CD8 ratio *(1 mark)*

Increased viral load *(1 mark)*

b *(1 mark for each correct answer, maximum 3 marks)* /3

HIV is from the retrovirus family *(1 mark)*

CD4 cells are involved in immune protection *(1 mark)*

HIV virus is able to enter into these cells via glycoproteins and chemokine co-receptors *(1 mark)*

The virus is able to replicate inside the cells *(1 mark)* leading to destruction and depletion of CD4 cells *(1 mark)*

c *(1 mark for each correct answer, maximum 3 marks)* `/3`
Fungal – *Pneumocystitis carinii (1 mark)*, *Cryptococcus*
(1 mark), *Aspergillus (1 mark)*, *Candida (1 mark)*
Protozoal – toxoplasmosis *(1 mark)*, cryptosporidiosis
(1 mark), leishmaniasis *(1 mark)*
Viral – cytomegalovirus *(1 mark)*, HSV *(1 mark)*, EBV
(1 mark), HPV *(1 mark)*
Bacteria – TB *(1 mark)*

d Nucleoside reverse transcriptase   `/3`
inhibitors – lamivudine *(1 mark)*
Non-nucleoside reverse transcriptase
inhibitors – nevirapine *(1 mark)*
Protease inhibitor – ritonavir *(1 mark)*

e *(1 mark for each correct answer, maximum 3 marks)* `/3`
Maintain good physical health *(1 mark)*
Maintain good mental health *(1 mark)*
Prevent virus transmission *(1 mark)*
Improve quality of life *(1 mark)*

Summary
Patients with HIV are increasingly being diagnosed at genitourinary medicine clinics on routine testing, however it is still common to find patients with atypical infections. Despite there being no cure for HIV, thanks to improvements in medical technology many patients are able to live normal healthy lives. Vaccine development has proved difficult due to the variability of the virus and unpredictable immune responses. Health promotion regarding prevention is vitally important.

6 a *(1 mark for each correct answer, maximum 3 marks)* `/3`
Night sweats *(1 mark)*
Arthralgia *(1 mark)*
Muscle aches *(1 mark)*
Vomiting *(1 mark)*
Diarrhoea *(1 mark)*
Jaundice *(1 mark)*
Abdominal pain *(1 mark)*

b *(maximum 1 mark for species, 1 mark for vector)* `/2`
Plasmodium falciparum (1 mark)
Plasmodium vivax (1 mark)
Plasmodium ovale (1 mark)

Plasmodium malariae (1 mark)
Female *Anopheles* mosquito *(1 mark)*

c *(1 mark for each correct answer, maximum 2 marks)* `/2`
Female mosquito becomes infected by gametocytes
(1 mark)
7–20 day maturation cycle producing sporozoites
(1 mark)
Reside in the mosquito's salivary gland *(1 mark)*
Infect human when bitten, and are taken up
by the liver where they reproduce *(1 mark)*

d *(1 mark for each correct answer, maximum 2 marks)* `/2`
Infected red cells become haemolysed *(1 mark)*
Dyserythropoiesis *(1 mark)*
Depletion of folate *(1 mark)*
Associated splenomegaly and sequestration *(1 mark)*

e *(maximum 1 mark)* `/1`
Cerebral malaria *(1 mark)*
Acute tubular necrosis *(1 mark)*
DIC *(1 mark)*
ARDS *(1 mark)*
Splenic rupture *(1 mark)*
Hypotensive shock *(1 mark)*

f Blood film to identify the parasite *(1 mark)* `/1`

g *(maximum 1 mark)* `/1`
Quinine *(1 mark)*
Chloroquine *(1 mark)*
Proguanil *(1 mark)*
Mefloquine *(1 mark)*
Fansidar *(1 mark)*
Doxycycline *(1 mark)*

h *(1 mark for each correct answer, maximum 2 marks)* `/2`
Cover up at night with long sleeves and trousers
(1 mark)
Mosquito net and repellents *(1 mark)*
Prophylactic medication *(1 mark)*

Summary

Malaria is endemic in and around the tropics with huge numbers of infections per year. Travellers to endemic areas need to be cautious and avoid insect bites by using repellents and mosquito nets, and anti-malarial prophylaxis should be taken. Signs and symptoms to be aware of are fever, night sweats, arthralgia, muscle aches, jaundice, abdominal pain, diarrhoea and vomiting.

7 a Mumps *(1 mark)* `/1`
  b Paramyxovirus *(1 mark)* `/1`
  c *(1 mark for each correct answer, maximum 3 marks)* `/3`
    Meningitis *(1 mark)*
    Epididymo-orchitis *(1 mark)*
    Pancreatitis *(1 mark)*
    Myocarditis *(1 mark)*
    Hepatitis *(1 mark)*
  d Supportive (encourage food and fluids, rest) *(1 mark)* `/2`
    Analgesia *(1 mark)*
  e *(1 mark for each correct answer, maximum 2 marks)* `/2`
    Immunosuppressed *(1 mark)*
    Radiotherapy *(1 mark)*
    Untreated malignancy *(1 mark)*
    Receipt of another live vaccine within last 3 weeks
      (1 mark)
    Allergy to excipient ingredients (e.g. gelatin) *(1 mark)*
    Children with acute febrile illness *(1 mark)*
    Receipt of an immunoglobulin injection in the
      last 3 months *(1 mark)*
    Pregnancy *(1 mark)*
  f Due to the decreased uptake of the MMR `/1`
    vaccine *(1 mark)*

Summary

Patients present with a headache, fever, and enlargement of the parotid glands. After the development of a vaccine mumps became rare. However, with the recent backlash against MMR, uptake of the vaccine has decreased and outbreaks of mumps are becoming increasingly frequent as herd immunity becomes less effective. Mumps is due to a paramyxovirus infection which is spread through direct contact, with an average peak period of infectivity averaging around 2–3 days before the beginning of parotitis.

8 a *(1 mark for each correct answer, maximum 3 marks)* `/3`
    Prolonged NG tube *(1 mark)*
    PPI *(1 mark)*
    Prolonged hospital/nursing home stay *(1 mark)*

Extremes of age *(1 mark)*

Repeated enemas (because these alter bowel flora)
(1 mark)

Overuse of broad-spectrum antibiotics *(1 mark)*

b Pseudo-membranous colitis *(1 mark)* `/1`

c *(1 mark for each correct answer, maximum 4 marks)* `/4`

Control antibiotic prescribing *(1 mark)*

Patient isolation *(1 mark)*

Infection control nurses *(1 mark)*

Environmental cleaning with chlorine disinfectant
(1 mark)

Hand hygiene and training *(1 mark)*

d *(1 mark for each correct answer, maximum 3 marks)* `/3`

Patient isolation *(1 mark)*

Review antibiotics under local hospital guidelines
(vancomycin/metronidazole) *(1 mark)*

Fluids *(1 mark)*

Repeat stool culture in 6 weeks' time *(1 mark)*

Summary

C. difficile presents with copious watery stool usually following a course of antibiotics in the elderly, infirm, or very young. *C. diff.* has become a major problem in hospitals. Patients who have long hospital stays and those who are nursing home residents have a greater risk of being colonised, and due to their weakened condition become susceptible to the disease. The problem occurs due to the overuse of broad-spectrum antibiotics which disrupt normal gut flora, allowing *Clostridium difficile* to over-colonise.

9 a *(1 mark for each correct answer, maximum 3 marks)* `/3`

Occur on lower leg above the medial malleolus
(1 mark)

Venous eczema *(1 mark)*

Brown pigmentation from haemosiderin *(1 mark)*

Varicose veins *(1 mark)*

Lipodermatosclerosis *(1 mark)*

Atrophie blanche *(1 mark)*

b *(1 mark for each correct answer, maximum 3 marks)* `/3`

Elderly *(1 mark)*

Hospitalised *(1 mark)*

Nursing home resident *(1 mark)*

Open wound *(1 mark)*
Contact with healthcare workers *(1 mark)*
c *(1 mark for each correct answer, maximum 3 marks)*   **/3**
Hand hygiene *(1 mark)*
Barrier nursing *(1 mark)*
Side room *(1 mark)*
Deep cleaning of room following discharge
     (1 mark)
d Nose *(1 mark)*   **/3**
Groin *(1 mark)*
Armpit *(1 mark)*

Summary

MRSA is a strain of *Staphylococcus aureus* which has multiple resistances including to methicillin. It may be a commensal organism on the patient's skin, but tends to cause infections in elderly patients with open wounds, when it becomes difficult to treat. Therefore all high-risk patients are screened when admitted to hospital, and patients are treated before surgery with nasal and body washes.

10 a *(1 mark for each correct answer, maximum 2 marks)*   **/2**
Epidemics occur when there is a minor
antigenic shift in the virus *(1 mark)*,
pandemics occur when there is a major
antigenic shift *(1 mark)*. Epidemics tend to be
more localised, whereas pandemics are more severe
and can be worldwide *(1 mark)*.
b *(1 mark for each correct answer, maximum 2 marks)*   **/2**
Blood-borne *(1 mark)*
Transplacental *(1 mark)*
Faeco-oral *(1 mark)*
Airborne *(1 mark)*
Droplet spread *(1 mark)*
Direct contact *(1 mark)*
c *(1 mark for each correct answer, maximum 3 marks)*   **/3**
Fever *(1 mark)*
Shivering *(1 mark)*
Generalised aches and pains *(1 mark)*
Severe headache *(1 mark)*
Sore throat *(1 mark)*
Dry cough *(1 mark)*

Rhinitis *(1 mark)*

Myalgia *(1 mark)*

d *(1 mark for each correct answer, maximum 3 marks)*   /3

All people over 65 *(1 mark)*

Healthcare workers *(1 mark)*

People under 65 who have a chronic health
  problem such as diabetes, chronic heart disease,
  chronic lung disease, chronic renal failure,
  immunosuppressed *(1 mark)*

Carers *(1 mark)*

Summary

There are two main types of influenza virus; A and B. B is typically associated with milder, localised outbreaks whereas A is associated with severe pandemics. Treatment is with bed rest, analgesia and antibiotics only for those patients with chronic renal, heart or lung diseases. Neuraminidase inhibitors may be used to shorten the duration of symptoms in the elderly and 'at risk' patients. Complications include the development of bacterial infections and pneumonia.

11 Dermatology

QUESTIONS

1 Ismail is a 2-year-old boy who is admitted with a skin rash to the paediatric department where you work.

   a Suggest four further questions you would ask about his rash.

     Mum and Dad say the rash has always been present on his face but it has got worse recently after they were given a puppy and is now present in the skin folds of his elbows and legs. On examination the flexor surfaces of elbows and knees are red and excoriated. There is some evidence of bleeding on these sites. **4 marks**

   b What diagnosis do you make? **1 mark**

   c Suggest three treatments you could initiate. **3 marks**

   d What two other medical problems can be associated with atopic skin conditions? **2 marks**

   e Mum and Dad are devastated by the diagnosis. Suggest one way in which you can reassure them. **1 mark**

2 Jason is 24. He comes to see the dermatologist complaining of patches of silvery white skin on the extensor aspect of his elbows that flake off.

   a What is the likely diagnosis? **1 mark**

   b Give two other sites you would examine. **2 marks**

   c Despite having always considered himself healthy, Jason also mentions he is troubled by knee pains. What diagnosis would you consider now? **1 mark**

   d Suggest one histological finding that a skin biopsy might show in this case. **1 mark**

Complete SAQs for Medical Finals By P. Stather et al, Published 2010 by Blackwell Publishing, ISBN: 978-1-4501-8928-6.

e Other than PUVA, name four methods of treating this condition. *4 marks*

f What is the risk of PUVA therapy? *1 mark*

3 Jamie is 17. Her GP has referred her to dermatology outpatients with severe acne.

a Give three features of the pathophysiology of acne. *3 marks*

b Which two areas of skin tend to be most affected by acne? *2 marks*

c Suggest two psychosocial problems Jamie may suffer from because of this. *2 marks*

d Suggest three treatments she may already have tried. *3 marks*

e What further treatment may the dermatologist be able to offer and give two potential side effects of this treatment *3 marks*

4 Mark is an 82-year-old ex-farmer. He is brought to see you by his daughter who is worried about a blemish on the side of his nose. You diagnose a basal cell carcinoma (BCC).

a What is the other name for a BCC? *1 mark*

b Suggest three groups of people who more commonly suffer from this condition. *3 marks*

c Give three features characteristic of a BCC. *3 marks*

d Give two options for treatment. *2 marks*

e Suggest two strategies you would advise patients to use to prevent this condition developing. *1 mark*

5 Sasha attends the GP surgery complaining of a small pea-sized nodule on her left shoulder that has appeared over the last few months. Sasha thinks it is a mole that she has caught on her bra strap because the middle of the mole is starting to appear nasty.

a What is a 'mole'? *1 mark*

b Other than squamous cell carcinoma give two differential diagnoses for a mole. *2 marks*

c When examining a patient, give four features you would comment on when describing a skin lesion. *4 marks*

d What other system would you need to examine? *1 mark*

e Suggest two groups of people who are more at risk of developing squamous cell carcinoma. *2 marks*

f Explain what a mole map is. *1 mark*

6 Tom is a 32-year-old builder. He is brought to his GP by his mother who is terrified that the mole on his arm is a malignant melanoma. She recently read a magazine article on melanomas and says he has all the features.

a Give five features of a malignant melanoma.   *5 marks*

b Which two sites of the body carry the worst
prognosis for malignant melanoma?   *2 marks*

c Give three ways you would manage a patient
with malignant melanoma.   *3 marks*

7 Beth is 17. She presents to her GP with dry cracked skin on her hands and wrists, which improves over the weekend. She has recently started college on a vocational course.

a What is the likely diagnosis?   *1 mark*

b Give three further questions you would ask
her to ascertain if your diagnosis is correct.   *3 marks*

c Suggest two careers known to have a high
incidence of causing these sort of problems.   *2 marks*

d By what two mechanisms can the dermatitis
be triggered?   *2 marks*

e Give three management strategies you could
advise for Beth.   *3 marks*

8 Muriel is 82, and she has been admitted to hospital by her GP. The district nurse has been dressing wounds on Muriel's legs for the last 5 months but has become concerned recently that the wounds were not showing any improvement. She has on this occasion noticed a spreading red patch on her leg, which is warm, although the ulcers appear to have not changed. Swabs for MRSA come back negative. Muriel is known to suffer from hypertension and raised cholesterol, with no other past history.

a What is the likely diagnosis?   *1 mark*

b What organism may be responsible for
the infection?   *1 mark*

c Assuming she has no drug allergies what
antibiotic treatment will you initiate until
sensitivities are known?   *2 marks*

d On reading the referral letter it transpires that
the wounds were due to ulcers caused by
varicose veins. What three other types of ulcer
are there?   *3 marks*

    e For each of the above types of ulcer identify
       which group of patients are most at risk.   *3 marks*
    f What two dermatological features may you see
      in a patient with varicose veins?   *2 marks*

9 A young mother brings her son to the GP surgery. She is concerned that he has chicken pox because 2 days ago he was playing with a child in the park who had a crusty scab on his face. Her own son now has a crusted lesion on his chin which is oozing yellow pus.

    a How do you know it is not chicken pox?   *1 mark*
    b You suspect that the lesion is due to impetigo.
      What advice will you give about the impetigo?   *1 mark*
    c Name one bacterial toxin implicated in
      impetigo infections.   *1 mark*
    d What medical treatment is required for impetigo?   *1 mark*
    e What is the incubation period for chicken pox?   *1 mark*
    f What is the virus responsible for causing
      chicken pox and shingles?   *1 mark*
    g How does shingles present differently to
      chicken pox?   *2 marks*
    h Why does shingles occur?   *1 mark*
    i What group of people are more likely to
      have shingles?   *1 mark*

10 You are working in the GP clinic. Your first patient is a 28-year-old football player who comes to see you complaining of recurrent 'athlete's foot'.

    a What is the organism responsible for causing this?   *1 mark*
    b Give one way of treating it.   *1 mark*
    c Later that day you see a second patient
      complaining of an intense itching and
      cream-coloured discharge from his penis.
      Give three differential diagnoses.   *3 marks*
    d What three further questions would you ask
      to ascertain the likely cause for this discharge?   *3 marks*
    e The swab you send away shows *Candida albicans,*
      more commonly known as thrush. Give two
      ways you would manage this.   *2 marks*

Dermatology

ANSWERS

1 a *(1 mark for each correct answer, maximum 4 marks)*   `/4`
Does it blanch? *(1 mark)*
Does it itch? *(1 mark)*
What is its distribution? *(1 mark)*
How long has it been there? *(1 mark)*
Any recent changes in washing powder, foods,
pets, etc? *(1 mark)*
Any known allergies? *(1 mark)*
Any family history of allergies or atopic
conditions? *(1 mark)*
Has Ismail had a fever recently? *(1 mark)*
Has Ismail been systemically unwell recently,
e.g. viral illness such as diarrhoea? *(1 mark)*
Is he well in himself, i.e. drinking, playing,
eating? *(1 mark)*
Has Ismail been wheezing or having any
breathing difficulties recently? *(1 mark)*
b Atopic eczema *(1 mark)*   `/1`
c *(1 mark for each correct answer, maximum 3 marks)*   `/3`
Liberal use of emollient creams and bath oils *(1 mark)*
Wet wrapping *(1 mark)*
Thorough drying of skin after bathing, especially
skin folds *(1 mark)*
Encourage Ismail not to scratch, and get his parents
to reward him for not scratching *(1 mark)*
Sparing use of steroid creams during flare-ups,
either topical or systemic *(1 mark)*
Trial of oral antihistamines to decrease itching *(1 mark)*
Avoid irritants, e.g. soap, perfumes *(1 mark)*
Suggest rehoming of the puppy *(1 mark)*
d Asthma *(1 mark)*   `/2`
Hayfever or allergic states *(1 mark)*
e *(maximum 1 mark)*   `/1`

Eczema is common in young children and most
 grow out of the condition as they grow up *(1 mark)*
Eczema is not contagious *(1 mark)*
Eczema is treatable *(1 mark)*

Summary

Eczema is a commonly seen problem in paediatrics. It may be very distressing for sufferers and their families so it is important to ensure they are well informed about managing their condition. Eczema is associated with increased serum IgE. Eczematous lesions may become secondarily infected with organisms such as *Staphylococcus aureus*.

2 a Psoriasis *(1 mark)* `/1`

  b *(1 mark for each correct answer, maximum 2 marks)* `/2`
    Nails *(1 mark)*
    Scalp *(1 mark)*
    Rest of skin (especially extensor surfaces) *(1 mark)*

  c Psoriatic arthritis *(1 mark)* `/1`

  d *(maximum 1 mark)* `/1`
    Irregular epidermal hyperplasia *(1 mark)*
    Absence of the granular cell layer *(1 mark)*
    Retention of nuclei in the horny layer *(1 mark)*
    Suprapapillary thinning *(1 mark)*
    Clubbing of rete pegs *(1 mark)*
    Leukocyte infiltration *(1 mark)*
    Epidermal pustulosis *(1 mark)*

  e *(1 mark for each correct answer, maximum 4 marks)* `/4`
    Moisturisers *(1 mark)*
    Tar *(1 mark)*
    Steroids *(1 mark)*
    Vitamin D analogues *(1 mark)*
    Methotrexate *(1 mark)*
    Retinoids *(1 mark)*
    Cyclosporin *(1 mark)*
    Immunomodulatory creams, e.g. tacrolimus *(1 mark)*
    Biological agents, e.g. etanercept *(1 mark)*

  f Increased risk of neoplastic skin lesions *(1 mark)* `/1`

Summary

Psoriasis is a debilitating condition that often runs in families. Sufferers may find that stress can induce or exacerbate the condition.

Nail changes seen in psoriasis include pitting and onycholysis. Plaques may form along scratch/trauma scars – this is called koebnerisation.

3 a *(1 mark for each correct answer, maximum 3 marks)* `/3`
Increased sebum excretion *(1 mark)*
Duct hyperkeratosis *(1 mark)*
Colonisation of the duct with bacteria *(1 mark)*
Release of inflammatory mediators *(1 mark)*

b *(1 mark for each correct answer, maximum 2 marks)* `/2`
Face *(1 mark)*
Back *(1 mark)*
Chest *(1 mark)*
Upper arms *(1 mark)*

c *(1 mark for each correct answer, maximum 2 marks)* `/2`
Embarrassment *(1 mark)*
Shame *(1 mark)*
Bullying *(1 mark)*
Depression *(1 mark)*
Lack of confidence *(1 mark)*

d *(1 mark for each correct answer, maximum 3 marks)* `/3`
Benzoyl peroxide topical creams *(1 mark)*
Antibiotics, topical and systemic *(1 mark)*
Oral contraceptive pill *(1 mark)*
Topical retinoids *(1 mark)*

e Isotretinoin (Roaccutane) *(1 mark)* `/3`
(maximum 2 marks for side-effects)
Derangement of LFTs and fasting lipids *(1 mark)*
Teratogenic effects on pregnancies *(1 mark)*
Depression *(1 mark)*
Muscle aches *(1 mark)*
Hair loss *(1 mark)*
Cracked lips *(1 mark)*
Dry skin *(1 mark)*
Nose bleeds *(1 mark)*
Photosensitivity *(1 mark)*

Summary

Acne is a very common complaint that typically affects teenagers. Although it causes no major damage to a patient's health it can be psychologically damaging to patients who may find they are stigmatized and bullied by others. It is important to offer them support as well as medical therapies.

4 a Rodent ulcer *(1 mark)* ⬚ /1

b *(1 mark for each correct answer, maximum 3 marks)* ⬚ /3
Elderly *(1 mark)*
Fair-skinned *(1 mark)*
History of sun exposure *(1 mark)*
Red-heads *(1 mark)*

c *(1 mark for each correct answer, maximum 3 marks)* ⬚ /3
Mainly (but not exclusively) occur on the face,
especially at side of nose or periorbital skin *(1 mark)*
May be flesh-coloured papules or plaques with superficial
dilated blood vessels over the surface *(1 mark)*
Raised pearly rolled edge *(1 mark)*
May be central necrosis with ulceration
or crusting *(1 mark)*
May be pigmented or cystic *(1 mark)*
May be locally invasive *(1 mark)*
Metastases are rare *(1 mark)*

d *(1 mark for each correct answer, maximum 2 marks)* ⬚ /2
Surgical excision *(1 mark)*
Cryotherapy *(1 mark)*
Radiotherapy *(1 mark)*
Medical therapy (Aldara/imiquimod cream for
superficial spreading BCCs) *(1 mark)*

e *(maximum 1 mark)* ⬚ /1
Stay out of sun at peak periods (between 11 a.m.
and 3 p.m.) *(½ mark)*
Wear a hat and sunglasses *(½ mark)*
Use sunscreen *(½ mark)*

Summary

Basal cell carcinoma is the most common form of skin tumour. It is an increasingly common phenomenon as more and more people have an increased sun exposure due to the increased number of foreign holidays. Although metastases are rare, local invasion can be very destructive.

5 a A mole (melanocytic naevus) is a benign ⬚ /1
overgrowth of melanocytes *(1 mark)*

b *(1 mark for each correct answer, maximum 2 marks)* ⬚ /2
Basal cell carcinoma *(1 mark)*
Seborrhoeic wart *(1 mark)*
Malignant melanoma *(1 mark)*

c *(1 mark for each correct answer, maximum 4 marks)* `/4`
Site *(1 mark)*
Size *(1 mark)*
Shape *(1 mark)*
Colour *(1 mark)*
Regularity/irregularity *(1 mark)*
Consistency *(1 mark)*
Any mass palpable below lesion *(1 mark)*
Discharge, i.e. pus or blood *(1 mark)*
If it is an isolated lesion or one of many *(1 mark)*
Nature of surrounding skin *(1 mark)*
Any recent change *(1 mark)*

d Lymphatic system looking for metastases, `/1`
i.e. examination of the lymph nodes *(1 mark)*

e *(1 mark for each correct answer, maximum 2 marks)* `/2`
People with a history of sun exposure *(1 mark)*
People who have had prolonged periods of
   immuno-suppressants (e.g. transplant patients)
   (1 mark)
Smokers *(1 mark)*
Patients who have received PUVA therapy *(1 mark)*
Wart virus in genital lesions *(1 mark)*

f Photographs of the whole body are taken and `/1`
used for comparison over time to look for new
lesions or growing ones *(1 mark)*

Summary

Squamous cell carcinomas may metastasise to regional lymph nodes. Tumours found on the lips and mouth are associated with smoking whereas those tumours found in the genital region are associated with the wart virus. All patients who have had one squamous cell carcinoma should be thoroughly examined for further lesions and advised about sun avoidance.

6 a *(1 mark for each correct answer, maximum 5 marks)* `/5`
Rapidly growing *(1 mark)*
Bleeding pigmented lesions *(1 mark)*
Asymmetry *(1 mark)*
Border irregularity *(1 mark)*
Colour variation *(1 mark)*
Diameter >6 mm *(1 mark)*
Halo of erythema *(1 mark)*

Ulceration *(1 mark)*
Persistent itching *(1 mark)*
Small 'satellite' lesions around the principal
  lesion *(1 mark)*
Regional lymphadenopathy *(1 mark)*
Metastases occur *(1 mark)*
b Head and neck *(1 mark)*   /2
Back of the arms *(1 mark)*
c *(1 mark for each correct answer, maximum 3 marks)*   /3
Surveillance photography of all moles *(1 mark)*
Referral to specialist *(1 mark)*
CT/MRI scan to check for metastasis *(1 mark)*
Excision with 2 cm margin (possibly with
  skin grafting) *(1 mark)*
Sun awareness *(1 mark)*
Self-examination and awareness *(1 mark)*
Regular examination of lymph nodes *(1 mark)*

Summary

It is vitally important that any suspicious-looking mole is further investigated. Any mole with more than three suspicious features should be
considered to be melanoma until proven otherwise. Treatment is via
surgical excision with a wide margin. Patients should also be monitored for signs of local recurrence or metastases for the next 5 years.

7 a Allergic contact dermatitis *(1 mark)*   /1
b *(1 mark for each correct answer, maximum 3 marks)*   /3
How long has this been happening? *(1 mark)*
Is the rash itchy? *(1 mark)*
What potential allergens has she had contact
  with? *(1 mark)*
Any idea what has caused it? *(1 mark)*
Ever had anything similar in the past, and if so
  what caused it then? *(1 mark)*
Any allergies of her own? *(1 mark)*
Any family history of allergies? *(1 mark)*
Does she suffer from asthma or hayfever? *(1 mark)*
c *(1 mark for each correct answer, maximum 2 marks)*   /2
Hairdressing *(1 mark)*
Building trade *(1 mark)*
Mechanic *(1 mark)*
Nursing *(1 mark)*

   d Direct irritation *(1 mark)*   `/2`
      Allergic reaction (type IV delayed hypersensitivity)
        (1 mark)
   e *(1 mark for each correct answer, maximum 3 marks)*   `/3`
      Avoid irritant substances *(1 mark)*
      Don't wear costume jewellery made of nickel as
        it could trigger a similar reaction *(1 mark)*
      Use of protective clothing such as gloves *(1 mark)*
      Emollient creams applied prior to contact with
        irritants to form a barrier *(1 mark)*
      Change of hobbies/careers *(1 mark)*

Summary

Type I hypersensitivity is an IgE-mediated response seen in ana-phylaxis; type II hypersensitivity is a cytotoxic, antibody-dependent reaction involving IgG or IgM; type III hypersensitivity is seen in immune complex diseases such as SLE and involves IgG and complement complexes. Type IV delayed hypersensitivity is a cell-mediated, antibody-independent reaction mediated by macrophages, natural killer cells and cytotoxic T-cells as seen in allergic contact dermatitis.

8 a Cellulitis *(1 mark)*   `/1`
   b *(maximum 1 mark)*   `/1`
      Staphylococcus species *(1 mark)*
      Streptococcus species *(1 mark)*
      Anaerobes *(1 mark)*
      Haemophilus influenzae (more rarely; seen in
        facial cellulitis usually) *(1 mark)*
   c *(1 mark for each correct answer, maximum 2 marks)*   `/2`
      Flucloxacillin *(1 mark)*
      Benzylpenicillin *(1 mark)*
      Metronidazole may be used if anaerobes
        suspected *(1 mark)*
   d Pressure sores (decubitus ulcers) *(1 mark)*   `/3`
      Arterial ulcers *(1 mark)*
      Neuropathic ulcers *(1 mark)*
   e Pressure sores – immobile, elderly, unconscious   `/3`
        patients *(1 mark)*
      Arterial ulcers – claudicants, smokers,
        hypertensives *(1 mark)*
      Neuropathic ulcers – diabetics, leprosy
        sufferers *(1 mark)*

f *(1 mark for each correct answer, maximum 2 marks)* `/2`
Venous eczema *(1 mark)*
Brown pigmentation from haemosiderin *(1 mark)*
Lipodermatosclerosis *(1 mark)*
Atrophie blanche (scarring white atrophy with
telangiectasia) *(1 mark)*
Thinning of skin *(1 mark)*
Loss of hair *(1 mark)*

Summary

Cellulitis most commonly occurs on the legs and feet but may in fact occur at any site. The organism may gain entry under the skin due to minor traumas such as abrasions, which are common in elderly people who are prone to falls. Ulcers also provide a means of entry for bacteria. Elderly people may often suffer from a delirium in association with their cellulitis and this will resolve after successful treatment.

9 a Incubation period is too short for chicken pox `/1`
(1 mark)
b *(maximum 1 mark)* `/1`
It is highly infectious – anyone who is
affected needs their own towels, plates,
cutlery, etc. so they do not spread the infection
(1 mark)
Children must stay off school for at least a
week *(1 mark)*
c *(maximum 1 mark)* `/1`
Staphylococcus aureus (1 mark)
Group A *Streptococcus (1 mark)*
d *(maximum 1 mark))* `/1`
Topical fusidic acid *(1 mark)*
Flucloxacillin *(1 mark)*
e 14–21 days *(1 mark)* `/1`
f Varicella zoster virus (VZV) *(1 mark)* `/1`
g Chicken pox has a prodromal flu-like period `/2`
and a widespread vesicular rash *(1 mark)*
The onset of shingles is usually heralded by
severe dermatomal pain and the rash will
have a dermatomal distribution *(1 mark)*
h Due to reactivation of latent VZV from dorsal `/1`
root and/or cranial nerve ganglia *(1 mark)*

i *(maximum 1 mark)* `/1`
Immunosuppressed patients *(1 mark)*
Elderly *(1 mark)*

Summary

Chicken pox is a common childhood illness. However, the small proportion of children who never develop it may require immunization in later life if they chose to enter careers involving healthcare. The incubation period for chicken pox is 14–21 days and may be accompanied by a prodromal period of flu like symptoms. Impetigo is highly infectious and is caused by staphylococcus aureus or streptococcus. There are two types; bullous and non-bullous. In both forms there is exudation and crusting.

10 a Tinea pedis *(1 mark)* `/1`
   b *(maximum 1 mark)* `/1`
      Topical antifungal cream, e.g. ketaconazole *(1 mark)*
      Oral antifungal therapy, e.g. clotrimazole *(1 mark)*
   c *Candida* infection *(1 mark)* `/3`
      Chlamydia (1 mark)
      Gonorrhoea *(1 mark)*
   d *(1 mark for each correct answer, maximum 3 marks)* `/3`
      Number of sexual partners *(1 mark)*
      If he practises safe sex – use of condoms *(1 mark)*
      If sexual partners have any symptoms *(1 mark)*
      Look for underlying predisposing conditions
         such as diabetes *(1 mark)*
   e *(1 mark for each correct answer, maximum 2 marks)* `/2`
      Advise loose-fitting cotton underwear and
         clothing *(1 mark)*
      Advise avoiding strongly perfumed washing
         products *(1 mark)*
      Prescribe an antifungal treatment *(1 mark)*
      Treat partner *(1 mark)*

Summary

Fungal infections are very common and typically patients will treat themselves. The classical appearance is of flaky skin, occurring in skin folds, and brittle, damaged nails. Treatment is either topical or systemic and patients are advised about the importance of good hygiene, especially in skin folds.

12 Ophthalmology
QUESTIONS

1 Eileen is 47. She is not very health conscious and only attended the opticians for an eye test because it was a special offer. Prior to this she hadn't been to the opticians for 6 years. Eileen's visual acuity tests normally. However, on examination of her fundus the optician notes cupping of the optic disc and decides to refer to the local hospital's ophthalmology department where a diagnosis of open-angle glaucoma is made.

   a Other than cupping of the optic disc name three clinical features found in open-angle glaucoma.   *3 marks*

   b Name three risk factors for developing open-angle glaucoma.   *3 marks*

   c What is the aim of medical management?   *1 mark*

   d Suggest two classes of drugs which can be used to achieve this and identify how they work.   *2 marks*

   e What are the two surgical options for treating open-angle glaucoma?   *2 marks*

   f What advice should Eileen be given?   *1 mark*

   g Suggest two ways of improving Eileen's compliance.   *2 marks*

2 Martha is admitted to A & E with persistent vomiting. On speaking with the doctor she also describes a visual disturbance and her right eye is clearly red.

   a What is the likely diagnosis?   *1 mark*

   b Why does visual loss occur in this condition?   *1 mark*

   c On examination (other than red eye) what two signs would be seen?   *2 marks*

   d Which group of patients does this condition typically occur in?   *1 mark*

   e What is the pathology behind the development of this condition?   *2 marks*

Complete SAQs for Medical Finals By P. Stather et al, Published 2010 by Blackwell Publishing, ISBN: 978-1-4501-8928-6.

f Give three ways you would manage this lady
initially to preserve her vision and make her
feel better. *3 marks*

3 Max is 73. He has diabetes, arthritis, angina and hypercholesterolaemia and has recently noticed that his vision has started to
deteriorate and he has become conscious of 'blots' in his vision.
You examine his eyes and note a decrease in visual acuity as
well as the presence of exudates and some new vessel formation
on fundoscopy.

   a What is your diagnosis? *1 mark*
   b Suggest two other visual problems diabetes
   can cause. *2 marks*
   c Identify the four classes of diabetic retinopathy
   and give one feature found in each class. *4 marks*
   d Which other common medical condition can
   cause retinopathy? *1 mark*
   e Give three ways of managing Max's condition. *3 marks*

4 Maureen is 48. She presents to her GP with a 2-day history of
inflammation of her left eye which is also watering.

   a Give five other questions you would ask to
   enable you to make a diagnosis. *5 marks*
   b Identify four important causes of red eye. *4 marks*
   c What is a dendritic ulcer and how is it treated? *2 marks*

5 Sophie, a 40-year-old lady, attends A & E complaining of a sudden
onset of peripheral visual loss in her left eye. She is very distressed
because she thinks she has had a stroke. After extensive questioning she admits that she had suffered from some bouts of flashing
lights in the last few weeks which is unusual for her. After examining Sophie you make a diagnosis of retinal detachment.

   a Other than trauma identify two types of retinal
   detachment and explain the pathology behind each. *4 marks*
   b Identify four other signs and symptoms of retinal
   detachment. *4 marks*
   c How is retinal detachment managed? *1 mark*
   d Other than a break in the retina itself, name
   one cause of retinal detachment. *1 mark*

6 Steven is 27. He presents to his GP complaining his eye has
been red for the last few days. On examination the GP finds no

evidence of any purulent discharge and so makes a diagnosis of episcleritis.

a Name two other clinical features of episcleritis. *2 marks*

b Although the condition is normally self-limiting, Steven is keen for you to prescribe something to help speed up the resolution. Suggest two medications you could consider prescribing. *2 marks*

c If Steven had a painful eye with a purulent discharge which diagnosis would you then consider? *1 mark*

d Give three clinical features for the above condition. *3 marks*

e Suggest one underlying condition you might suspect. *1 mark*

f How will you treat Steven now? *1 mark*

7 Kirsty is 14. She comes from a family which has an extensive history of retinitis pigmentosa and Kirsty herself is affected by the condition.

a What are the four main symptoms of retinitis pigmentosa? *4 marks*

b Which three non-hereditary conditions may mimic the symptoms of retinitis pigmentosa? *3 marks*

c Other than pigmentation around the fundus give two features you might see on fundoscopy. *2 marks*

d Suggest two psychosocial problems Kirsty may suffer from. *2 marks*

e Give three services and voluntary organizations Kirsty may require assistance from. *3 marks*

8 Howard is 84. He arrives at the ophthalmology outpatient department with his daughter. She took him to see his GP recently because she was concerned that he was no longer able to see well enough to do his favourite hobby of model making. On examination the GP noted decreased visual acuity and found it difficult to elicit the red reflex in the left eye.

a What do you suspect the likely diagnosis to be? *1 mark*

b How is this condition broadly subdivided? *1 mark*

c Give two other features which are important to examine for or ask about. *2 marks*

d How is this condition commonly treated? *1 mark*

e Identify three systemic disorders that can cause this condition. *3 marks*

f Identify two risk factors that can cause this condition. *2 marks*

9 Sybil is 84. She has always been active and independent but has recently had a number of small bumps in her car. Concerned she needed new glasses she went to see her optician who felt she may be developing Age Related Macular Degeneration (ARMD).

   a Which area of vision does ARMD typically affect?   *1 mark*

   b What are the two types of macular degeneration and how do you distinguish between the two?   *4 marks*

   c Give three clinical features of ARMD.   *3 marks*

   d What are Drusen?   *1 mark*

   e What is the prognosis of both forms of ARMD?   *2 marks*

   f Give two management methods you would consider for ARMD.   *2 marks*

10 Mark is 17. He is brought to A & E by the police who have found him slumped unconscious in a pool of his own blood. He appears to have a broken rib, multiple bruises and a heavily bruised and swollen left eye and surrounding structures. The police believe he has been in a fight.

   a What will be your initial priority in his management?   *4 marks*

   b Later, after ordering an x-ray of Mark's face a diagnosis of blowout fracture is made. Give two features (other than bone fractures) that may be seen on the x-ray that draw you to this diagnosis.   *2 marks*

   c Name four of the bones that make up the orbit.   *4 marks*

   d Which nerve that runs along the floor of the orbit may be damaged by this fracture?   *1 mark*

      What is the result of damage to this nerve?   *1 mark*

Ophthalmology

ANSWERS

1 a Visual field loss *(1 mark)* /3
  Intraocular pressure usually raised *(1 mark)*
  Open anterior chamber. *(1 mark)*
  b *(1 mark for each correct answer, maximum 3 marks)* /3
  Genetic – it is more common in first-degree
    relatives *(1 mark)*
  Increasing age *(1 mark)*
  Diabetes mellitus *(1 mark)*
  Myopia *(1 mark)*
  Black race *(1 mark)*
  c To lower intraocular pressure *(1 mark)* /1
  d *(1 mark for each correct answer, maximum 2 marks)* /2
  Beta-blocker eye drop *(½ mark)* – topical aqueous
    humour suppression *(½ mark)*
  Carbonic anhydrase enzyme inhibitors
    (½ mark) – inhibit aqueous humour production
    (½ mark)
  Alpha-adrenergic receptors *(½ mark)* – reduce
    aqueous humour production *(½ mark)*
  Prostaglandin analogues *(½ mark)* – enhancement of
    aqueous outflow *(½ mark)*
  e Laser surgery – induces changes at the trabecular /2
    meshwork that lead to a lower intraocular
    pressure *(1 mark)*
  Trabeculectomy – creates an opening in the
    anterior chamber angle for drainage *(1 mark)*
  f *(maximum 1 mark)* /1
  Importance of looking after her health *(1 mark)*
  That her first-degree relatives are now eligible
    for free eye tests as they have an increased
    risk of developing glaucoma *(1 mark)*
  g *(1 mark for each correct answer, maximum 2 marks)* /2
  Offer advice about the risk of not complying
    with medication *(1 mark)*

Offer information about side-effects *(1 mark)*

Prescribe drugs according to lowest side-effect
profile *(1 mark)*

Regular follow up appointments with lots of
encouragement *(1 mark)*

Simplest dosing possible, such as once per day *(1 mark)*

Summary

Open-angle glaucoma is the most common type of glau-coma, affecting 1% of those over 40 and 10% of those over 80. Aqueous humour drains through the trabecular mesh-work which over time undergoes changes which impair drain-age. This causes a rise in intraocular pressure, which damages the optic nerve and disc. Relatives of people with glaucoma are offered free screening due to their increased risk of having the condition.

2 a Acute-angle closure glaucoma *(1 mark)* `/1`

  b Corneal oedema *(1 mark)* `/1`

  c Loss of red reflex *(1 mark)* `/2`
Oval, non-reactive pupil *(1 mark)*

  d Hypermetropic patients *(1 mark)* `/1`

  e *(1 mark for each correct answer, maximum 2 marks)* `/2`
There is crowding of the anterior chamber angle
(1 mark) which means aqueous humour is
prevented from accessing the trabecular
meshwork *(1 mark)* thus increasing the
intraocular pressure *(1 mark)*

  f *(1 mark for each correct answer, maximum 3 marks)* `/3`
Beta-blockers – aqueous suppressant *(1 mark)*
Acetazolamide – aqueous suppressant *(1 mark)*
Analgesics *(1 mark)*
Anti-emetics *(1 mark)*

Summary

Acute-angle closure glaucoma occurs where the aqueous humour fails to pass through the pupil, causing raised pressure in the anterior chamber. This is usually an acute rise, which may either resolve spontaneously, or cause severe permanent visual loss. Patients with acute-angle closure glaucoma therefore need urgent attention when they present.

3 a Diabetic retinopathy *(1 mark)* — `/1`

  b *(1 mark for each correct answer, maximum 2 marks)* — `/2`
    Cataract *(1 mark)*
    Retinal vascular occlusions *(1 mark)*
    Extraocular muscle palsy *(1 mark)*

  c Background *(½ mark)* – microaneurysms; dot and — `/4`
    blot haemorrhages; exudates *(½ mark)*
    Preproliferative *(½ mark)* – cotton wool spots; venous
    beading, loops and doubling *(½ mark)*
    Proliferative *(½ mark)* – new vessels at the disc and
    elsewhere *(½ mark)*
    Maculopathy *(½ mark)* – microaneurysms;
    haemorrhages; exudates; oedema at the
    macula *(½ mark)*

  d Hypertension *(1 mark)* — `/1`

  e *(1 mark for each correct answer, maximum 3 marks)* — `/3`
    Excellent diabetic control *(1 mark)*
    Excellent blood pressure control *(1 mark)*
    Regular screening and follow up in appropriate
    out patient clinic *(1 mark)*
    Fluorescein angiography to identify vessels with
    potential to treat *(1 mark)*
    Laser treatment *(1 mark)*

Summary

Retinopathy occurs in virtually all type 1 diabetics within 20 years of diagnosis. It is therefore screened for as part of the diabetic screening programme. The visual loss is usually caused by maculopathy or vitreous haemorrhage. Patients with early changes are offered laser therapy and those with severe changes may require vitrectomy. Retinopathy is also seen in patients with uncontrolled hypertension.

4 a *(1 mark for each correct answer, maximum 5 marks)* — `/5`
    Any discomfort? *(1 mark)*
    Any history of trauma? *(1 mark)*
    Any visual disturbance? *(1 mark)*
    Any headache? *(1 mark)*
    Any nausea/vomiting? *(1 mark)*
    Any problems in the right eye? *(1 mark)*
    Any past medical/ocular history? *(1 mark)*

Any itching? *(1 mark)*

Any discharge? *(1 mark)*

Any recent close contacts with anything
similar? *(1 mark)*

b *(1 mark for each correct answer, maximum 4 marks)* **/4**

Conjunctivitis: infections (bacterial, viral), allergic
(1 mark)

Acute-angle closure glaucoma *(1 mark)*

Acute iritis *(1 mark)*

Trauma: subconjunctival haemorrhage, corneal
abrasion, corneal foreign body, penetrating
injury *(1 mark)*

Keratitis *(1 mark)*

Scleritis *(1 mark)*

Episcleritis *(1 mark)*

Subconjunctival haemorrhage *(1 mark)*

c Ulcer caused by herpes simplex virus *(1 mark)* **/2**

Treat with topical acyclovir ointment *(1 mark)*

Follow up in ophthalmology clinic.

Summary

A common cause of red eye (especially in children) is conjunctivitis. Conjunctivitis may be due to allergies or infection by either bacteria or viruses. Simple topical treatments will usually provide relief but it is vital to take the opportunity to reiterate basic rules of health promotion to prevent the spread of the disease. Patients should be reminded about the necessity of hand washing after they have used their eye drops and advised to avoid touching the eye as much as possible.

5 a *(1 mark for each correct answer, maximum 4 marks)* **/4**

Tractional *(1 mark)* – the retina is pulled off by
membranes which are growing across its surface
(e.g. advanced diabetic retinopathy) *(1 mark)*

Exudative *(1 mark)* – breakdown of the blood–retinal
barrier allow fluid to accumulate in the
subretinal space *(1 mark)*

Rhegmatogenous *(1 mark)* – degenerative changes in
the neurosensory retina create a hole through
which fluid from the vitreous humour passes into
the subretinal space leading to detachment *(1 mark)*

b *(1 mark for each correct answer, maximum 4 marks)* `/4`
Peripheral field loss initially *(1 mark)*
Floaters/flashing lights *(1 mark)*
Description of visual loss as similar to 'curtain coming across' *(1 mark)*
Loss of red reflex *(1 mark)*
Loss of central vision at a later stage *(1 mark)*
Detached retina appears grey on fundoscopy *(1 mark)*
c Vitrectomy to remove traction of the vitreous *(1 mark)* `/1`
d *(maximum 1 mark)* `/1`
Proliferative diabetic retinopathy *(1 mark)*
Uveitis *(1 mark)*
Intraocular tumours *(1 mark)*

Summary

Most cases of retinal detachment are due to a tear in the retina. This happens when the vitreous exerts traction on the retina. Surgical options include vitrectomy, but if the retina has been detached for more than 2 days then central vision is impaired. Reattachment may occur due to proliferation of retinal scar tissue.

6 a *(1 mark for each correct answer, maximum 2 marks)* `/2`
Inflammation is superficial and bright red *(1 mark)*
Pain is absent to mild *(1 mark)*
Hyperaemia can be segmental or diffuse *(1 mark)*
Visual disturbance is rare *(1 mark)*
Systemic disease is only rarely associated with episcleritis *(1 mark)*
b Weak topical steroids *(1 mark)* `/2`
NSAIDs *(1 mark)*
c *(maximum 1 mark)* `/1`
Scleritis *(1 mark)*
Conjunctivitis *(1 mark)*
d *(1 mark for each correct answer, maximum 3 marks)* `/3`
Presence of associated systemic disease *(1 mark)*
Inflammation involves full thickness of the sclera *(1 mark)*
Large, deep blood vessels are seen to be swollen when examined with the slit lamp *(1 mark)*
Inflammation involves the whole circumference of the anterior segment *(1 mark)*

Scleral thinning *(1 mark)*
Corneal thinning *(1 mark)*
Perforation *(1 mark)*
  e *(maximum 1 mark)*   /1
Systemic lupus erythematosus *(1 mark)*
Rheumatoid arthritis *(1 mark)*
Herpes zoster ophthalmicus *(1 mark)*
  f *(maximum 1 mark)*   /1
Steroids *(1 mark)*
NSAIDs *(1 mark)*
Immunosuppressive therapy *(1 mark)*

Summary

The most important way to differentiate between episcleritis and scleritis is that scleritis is associated with pain, although it is much less common than episcleritis. Scleritis is a feature of a number of systemic conditions such as SLE and rheumatoid arthritis, and patients presenting with scleritis should be questioned about systemic symptoms.

7 a Nyctalopia (night blindness) *(1 mark)*   /4
Decreased peripheral vision *(1 mark)*
Decreased central vision *(1 mark)*
Glare (from cataract) *(1 mark)*
  b *(1 mark for each correct answer, maximum 3 marks)*   /3
Trauma *(1 mark)*
Drugs such as chlorpromazine *(1 mark)*
Retinal detachment surgery *(1 mark)*
Infections such as syphilis or rubella *(1 mark)*
Previous occlusion of retinal artery or vein *(1 mark)*
  c *(1 mark for each correct answer, maximum 2 marks)*   /2
Narrowing of the retinal arterioles giving a 'waxy'
    appearance *(1 mark)*
'Bone spicule' pigment clumping in mid periphery of
    retina *(1 mark)*
Cataract *(1 mark)*
Cystoid macular oedema *(1 mark)*
  d *(1 mark for each correct answer, maximum 2 marks)*   /2
Depression *(1 mark)*
Being stigmatized or bullied *(1 mark)*
Lack of confidence *(1 mark)*
Low self esteem and low self worth *(1 mark)*

   e *(1 mark for each correct answer, maximum 3 marks)*   /3
      School psychologist *(1 mark)*
      Classroom assistant *(1 mark)*
      Special needs schooling *(1 mark)*
      Social Services *(1 mark)*
      Benefits Agency *(1 mark)*
      Royal National Institute for the Blind *(1 mark)*
      Peer support groups *(1 mark)*
      Guide Dog Association *(1 mark)*

Summary

Retinitis pigmentosa is an inherited primary retinal degeneration, which affects the rods more than the cones. It initially presents with night blindness in childhood, and there is a progressive visual field loss leading to tunnel vision.

8 a Cataract *(1 mark)*   /1
   b Senile cataract *(1½ mark)*   /1
      Congenital or infantile cataract *(1½ mark)*
   c *(1 mark for each correct answer, maximum 2 marks)*   /2
      Glare from lights *(1 mark)*
      Monocular diplopia *(1 mark)*
      Relative afferent papillary defect *(1 mark)*
      Change in refraction (e.g. recently needing new
         glasses) *(1 mark)*
      Surgical removal of cataract and replacement with
         artificial lens *(1 mark)*
      Diabetes mellitus *(1 mark)*
   d Corticosteroid therapy *(1 mark)*   /1
   e *(1 mark for each correct answer, maximum 3 marks)*   /3
      Atopy *(1 mark)*
      Galactosaemia *(1 mark)*
      Hypocalcaemia *(1 mark)*
      Dystrophia myotonica *(1 mark)*
   f *(1 mark for each correct answer, maximum 2 marks)*   /2
      Topical steroid use *(1 mark)*
      Recurrent uveitis *(1 mark)*
      History of blunt or perforating trauma *(1 mark)*
      High myopia *(1 mark)*
      Ionising irradiation *(1 mark)*
      High exposure to ultraviolet light *(1 mark)*

Summary

Surgical correction of cataracts is very common. It may be performed under local anaesthetic. Most patients benefit from surgery, although the prognosis is poorer in those with systemic disease, and the surgery may result in loss of vision, glaucoma, amblyopia, strabismus, or retinal detachment.

9 a Central visual field *(1 mark)* /1

b Dry *(1 mark)* – slowly progressive deterioration of vision *(1 mark)* /4

Wet *(1 mark)* – There is new growth of abnormally located blood vessels underneath the retina causes sudden visual loss by haemorrhage or leakage of fluid *(1 mark)*

c *(1 mark for each correct answer, maximum 3 marks)* /3

Progressive, gradual loss of central loss of vision *(1 mark)*

Reading difficulty *(1 mark)*

Difficulty recognising distant objects *(1 mark)*

Distortion of straight lines *(1 mark)*

d Drusen are small yellow deposits commonly seen on the macula *(1 mark)* /1

e Dry – slow deterioration with minimal visual loss *(1 mark)* /2

Wet – marked deterioration occurs in 75% of patients within the first 3 years *(1 mark)*

f *(1 mark for each correct answer, maximum 2 marks)* /2

High-dose antioxidant vitamins *(1 mark)*

Possible registration as blind or visually impaired *(1 mark)*

Laser therapy for wet ARMD *(1 mark)*

Antivascular endothelial growth factor drugs such as Lucentis, Macugen and Avastin given as injections into the vitreous cavity of the eye *(1 mark)*

Summary

Age-related macular degeneration is the commonest cause of being registered blind in the western world. It appears as small yellow spots called Drusen or colloid bodies around the macula, with pigment speckling. There is often retinal atrophy resulting in the underlying larger choroidal vessels being visualised. Antivascular endothelial growth factor can only be used for the treatment of wet ARMD.

10 a *(1 mark for each correct answer, maximum 4 marks)*   /4
   Airway *(1 mark)*
   Breathing *(1 mark)*
   Circulation *(1 mark)*
   Stabilisation of Cervical spine *(1 mark)*
   Disability (neurological) *(1 mark)*
   Everything else (bones, etc.) *(1 mark)*
b Sinus fluid level due to haemorrhage *(1 mark)*   /2
   Teardrop sign – prolapse of orbital tissues into
      the maxillary sinus *(1 mark)*
c *(1 mark for each correct answer, maximum 4 marks)*   /4
   Frontal *(1 mark)*
   Maxilla *(1 mark)*
   Ethmoid *(1 mark)*
   Sphenoid *(1 mark)*
   Zygomatic *(1 mark)*
   Lacrimal *(1 mark)*
d Infraorbital nerve *(1 mark)*   /2
   Damage leads to altered sensation of the cheek *(1 mark)*

Summary

Ocular trauma is a common presentation in A & E. A thorough examination should be conducted to ensure there are no foreign bodies (such as glass) within the eye or under the eyelid and that there is no internal damage due to blunt trauma. Examination should be conducted using an ophthalmoscope and slit lamp.

13 Psychiatry

QUESTIONS

1 Rupert, a 36-year-old man, has been brought in to see you by his wife, who says that he does not seem himself. He believes he has been put onto this earth by God to do good, and that he is communicating with Jesus. He has also been sleeping less, and appears to be hyperactive, having lots of energy, and ideas.

   a What diagnosis do you suspect?   *1 mark*
   b Give three other symptoms of this condition.   *3 marks*
   c What two types of delusions may occur in this condition?   *2 marks*
   d Apart from lithium, name two other drugs that may help with this condition.   *2 marks*
   e Give two common side-effects of lithium.   *2 marks*

2 Prudence, a 66-year-old lady, has come to see you in the GP surgery. She has recently lost her husband, and feels very low. She has stopped going out, and feels she can no longer cope with life, although denies any suicidal ideation.

   a What are the three core symptoms of depression?   *3 marks*
   b State two other physical symptoms of depression.   *2 marks*
   c Give four blood tests you would do in this case.   *4 marks*
   d Give three different classes of antidepressants.   *3 marks*

3 Ursula, a 42-year-old lady, has come into A & E having taken an overdose of 100 paracetamol tablets 30 minutes previously. She is currently conscious and tearful, and her observations are normal.

   a Give three epidemiological risk factors for suicide.   *3 marks*
   b State three ways of determining the severity of her suicidal intent.   *3 marks*
   c Give four aspects of your management of this lady.   *4 marks*

Complete SAQs for Medical Finals By P. Stather et al, Published 2010 by Blackwell Publishing, ISBN: 978-1-4501-8928-6.

4 Paul, a 20-year-old maths student, has come to see you because he has been hearing voices talking about him, and is finding it difficult to sleep because of this.

   a Give three further questions you would ask him regarding the voices.   *3 marks*

   b State three further questions would you ask him.   *3 marks*

   c He tells you that the voices have been telling him to kill his parents, and you decide to admit him. Give one example of a typical and one example of an atypical antipsychotic that may be used in his treatment.   *2 marks*

   d List three side-effects of antipsychotics.   *3 marks*

5 Richard, a 33-year-old man, has come to see you in the GP surgery. He wants to be admitted to hospital for a detoxification programme as he has been drinking excessively throughout his life, drinking at least a bottle of vodka a day for the past 3 months, and says he no longer wants to carry on this way.

   a What are the four CAGE questions?   *4 marks*

   b Give four questions you would ask someone to determine if they were suffering from alcohol dependency.   *4 marks*

   c What is the name given to the condition he may develop if he suddenly stops consuming alcohol?   *1 mark*

   d How many units of alcohol are in i) a pint ii) a standard glass of wine iii) a shot of spirits?   *3 marks*

   e What is the recommended number of units per week for a man and a woman?   *2 marks*

6 Lawrence, a 51-year-old man, was in the pub as usual when he felt a pain in his abdomen. He went home to 'sleep it off' but has now come in and been admitted with severe epigastric pain radiating to his back. Two days after admission his behaviour becomes bizarre, and he says he is seeing things flying around his bed. He has no history of psychosis.

   a What is the likely cause of the abdominal pain and why?   *2 marks*

   b Give three other causes of this condition.   *3 marks*

   c Why is he seeing things flying around his bed?   *1 mark*

   d Apart from hallucinations, give three other symptoms of this condition.   *3 marks*

e State one medication that can be used to
control the symptoms. *1 mark*

7 Olivia, a 25-year-old lady, has come to see you in your GP surgery for the OCP. You notice that she appears very thin, and ask
her about her eating habits. You also weigh her and notice that
despite being 1.6 m tall, she weighs only 44 kg.
  a Give three of the diagnostic criteria for
  anorexia nervosa. *3 marks*
  b Apart from restricting food consumption, give
  three other methods this patient may use to
  avoid weight gain. *3 marks*
  c Calculate her BMI. *1 mark*
  d State four other signs and symptoms she may have. *4 marks*

8 You are working as a GP and have been asked to come out
for a home visit to see Nicholas, a 27-year-old man. His wife
phoned the surgery saying that her husband is having increasing difficulty leaving the house. He repeatedly checks that all
the windows and locks are fastened, and often returns to the
house early. Further questioning reveals that he feels very anxious when out of the house, and complains of feeling physically
unwell, with palpitations and sweating.
  a Give two possible diagnoses. *2 marks*
  b Give four other physical symptoms of anxiety
  disorders. *4 marks*
  c Name two different types of medication that
  may be used for this condition. *2 marks*
  d Apart from medication, give two treatment
  options that are available for this man. *2 marks*

9 Neil, an 80-year-old man, has been admitted to the elderly psychiatric ward suffering from severe dementia, and his wife is
unable to cope with his behaviour.
  a Please define dementia. *3 marks*
  b What are the three most common types of
  dementia? *3 marks*
  c When a patient is admitted with an acute
  confusional state, what two other common
  causes may there be for this? (2 mark)
  d Give two options for the further long-term care of
  Neil in the community. *2 marks*

10 Mary, a 72-year-old lady, has become more forgetful over the past year. She was found by the police last week wandering around the town centre by herself, and couldn't remember her way home. When you see her she scores 18/30 on the MMSE.

   a Below what MMSE score is the patient said to have dementia, if recorded on repeated occasions?   *1 mark*

   b What are the two pathological changes found on CT of a patient with Alzheimer's dementia?   *2 marks*

   c Suggest four routine blood tests you would request for this patient to check for other causes of dementia, and why?   *4 marks*

   d Give two options for the treatment of Alzheimer's dementia, with regard to medication.   *2 marks*

   e Describe three aspects of your long-term management of this patient.   *3 marks*

11 Penelope, a 67-year-old lady, has been admitted to A & E with deterioration in her functioning. She has been unable to cope at home, and was found by her daughter having left her cooker on and burnt her dinner, which was still on the hob. You dip-test her urine, and diagnose a UTI, causing delirium.

   a Please define delirium.   *3 marks*

   b Give three common causes of delirium.   *3 marks*

   c State four ways in which you can differentiate between delirium and dementia.   *4 marks*

   d It is found that Penelope is suffering from mild dementia as well, and requires some home help. Suggest three types of assistance that can be put in place for her.   *3 marks*

Psychiatry

ANSWERS

1 a *(maximum 1 mark)*　　　　　　　　　　　　　　$\boxed{/1}$
　　Bipolar affective disorder *(1 mark)*
　　Mania *(1 mark)*

b *(1 mark for each correct answer, maximum 3 marks)*　$\boxed{/3}$
　　Elevated mood *(1 mark)*
　　Increased spending *(1 mark)*
　　Increased libido *(1 mark)*
　　Increased appetite *(1 mark)*
　　Easily distracted *(1 mark)*
　　Easily agitated *(1 mark)*

c Auditory hallucinations *(1 mark)*, which are often　$\boxed{/2}$
　　　grandiose
　　Delusions of reference *(1 mark)*

d *(1 mark for each correct answer, maximum 2 marks)*　$\boxed{/2}$
　　Sodium valproate *(1 mark)*
　　Carbamazepine *(1 mark)*
　　Chlorpromazine *(1 mark)*
　　Olanzapine *(1 mark)*
　　Quetiapine *(1 mark)*

e *(1 mark for each correct answer, maximum 2 marks)*　$\boxed{/2}$
　　Tremor *(1 mark)*
　　Thinning of hair *(1 mark)*
　　Acne *(1 mark)*
　　Weight gain *(1 mark)*
　　Diabetes insipidus *(1 mark)*

Summary

Bipolar disorder usually presents with both low and elevated mood at different times, however it can occur with purely manic episodes and no depression. The typical symptoms are reduced sleep but no fatigue, increased appetite, weight loss, psychomotor acceleration, an increased drive in work and pleasure activities, and increased libido. People suffering from mania tend to wear bright clothing, are untidy, hyperactive, indiscreet, have a flight of ideas, and appear euphoric. There is often impaired concentration, and a lack of insight.

2 a Low mood for more than 2 weeks *(1 mark)* <u>/3</u>
    Anhedonia *(1 mark)*
    Fatigue/lethargy *(1 mark)*

  b *(1 mark for each correct answer, maximum 2 marks)* <u>/2</u>
    Sleep disturbance *(1 mark)* typically early morning
      wakening
    Loss of appetite *(1 mark)*
    Weight loss *(1 mark)*
    Loss of libido *(1 mark)*

  c *(1 mark for each correct answer, maximum 4 marks)* <u>/4</u>
    FBC *(1 mark)*
    U+E *(1 mark)*
    TFT *(1 mark)*
    Vitamin B12 *(1 mark)*
    Folate *(1 mark)*
    Glucose *(1 mark)*

  d *(1 mark for each correct answer, maximum 3 marks)* <u>/3</u>
    Tricyclics *(1 mark)*
    SSRIs *(1 mark)*
    SNRIs *(1 mark)*
    MAOIs *(1 mark)*

Summary

Depression is a very common condition, and can occur at any time in life. It can be classified as mild, involving two core symptoms and two other symptoms, moderate, involving two core symptoms and three or four other symptoms, or severe, involving all three core symptoms and four other symptoms. Depression may cause sleep disturbance with early morning wakening, loss of appetite and weight, and slowness. Patients often feel worse in the mornings, and have a loss of interest in pleasure activities, as well as a loss of libido, and occasionally constipation. The patient may appear neglected and sad, having decreased gestures, poverty of speech, hesitancy, irritability, and have morbid thoughts, feelings of hopelessness, and sometimes delusions or hallucinations.

3 a *(1 mark for each correct answer, maximum 3 marks)* <u>/3</u>
    Male (*1 mark*)
    Elderly *(1 mark)*
    Unemployed *(1 mark)*

Low socio-economic status *(1 mark)*
Previous psychiatric treatment *(1 mark)*
Living alone/homeless *(1 mark)*
b *(1 mark for each correct answer, maximum 3 marks)* `/3`
Whether she wished to die *(1 mark)*
If she wrote a note or will *(1 mark)*
Amount of attempt planning *(1 mark)*
Violence of method *(1 mark)*
If she still wishes to die *(1 mark)*
c *(1 mark for each correct answer, maximum 4 marks)* `/4`
Gastric lavage *(1 mark)*
Activated charcoal *(1 mark)* (activated charcoal and
gastric lavage are only used as treatment if the
overdose has been taken within the last hour)
Bloods *(1 mark)* (paracetamol and salicylate levels,
LFT, FBC, INR, ethanol)
Parvolex *(1 mark)*
Refer to psychiatry team *(1 mark)*

Summary

It is vitally important that suicide risk is assessed in every patient who attends with a psychiatric illness, particularly depression, or when a suicide attempt has been made. Significant predictors of risk are premeditation, taking precautions to avoid discovery, carrying out the attempt alone, making no attempts to obtain help, using a dangerous or violent method, and writing a suicide note or will. A previous history of self-harm, being male, over 45, having other psychiatric problems, being socially isolated, having physical co-morbidities, and unemployed are other risk factors.

4 a Content *(1 mark)* (are they telling him to hurt `/3`
himself or others?)
3rd and 2nd person hallucinations? *(1 mark)*
Running commentary? *(1 mark)*
Does it feel like the voice is your own thoughts
aloud, or a different person speaking? *(1 mark)*
Does he know who the voices are? *(1 mark)*
b Hallucinations in other sensory modalities? *(1 mark)* `/3`
Delusions (anyone out to get you, anyone
controlling you)? *(1 mark)*
Thought insertion/withdrawal/broadcast? *(1 mark)*
Change of mood? *(1 mark)*
Problems with memory? *(1 mark)*

Delusions of reference? *(1 mark)*
c Atypical – olanzapine, quetiapine, risperidone   /2
     (1 mark for any of these)
     Typical – chlorpromazine, haloperidol, flupenthixol
     (1 mark for any of these)
d *(1 mark for each correct answer, maximum 3 marks)*   /3
     Weight gain *(1 mark)*
     Dry mouth *(1 mark)*
     Muscle rigidity *(1 mark)*
     Tremor *(1 mark)*
     Extrapyramidal side-effects *(1 mark)*

Summary

Out of all patients having a first episode of schizophrenia 20% make a complete recovery, 20% have a recurrent acute illness, 20% have a chronic condition with acute episodes, 20% are chronic with an insidious onset, and 10–15% commit suicide.

Schneider's first rank symptoms of schizophrenia are: hearing thoughts spoken aloud; third person hallucinations; hallucinations in the form of a commentary; somatic hallucinations; thought withdrawal; thought insertion; thought broadcast; delusional perception; and feelings or actions being experienced as though made by external agents.

5 a Ever felt you should Cut down on alcohol? *(1 mark)*   /4
     Do you get Annoyed about people asking you about
       drinking? *(1 mark)*
     Do you feel Guilty about using alcohol? *(1 mark)*
     Do you need an Eye opener? *(1 mark)*
  b *(1 mark for each correct answer, maximum 4 marks)*   /4
     Have you felt that you should cut down on your
       drinking? *(1 mark)*
     Do you ever drink before driving or in hazardous
       situations? *(1 mark)*
     Is someone in your family concerned about your
       drinking? *(1 mark)*
     Have you ever had any blackouts or medical
       problems because of drinking? *(1 mark)*
     Have you ever been absent from work or lost a
       job because of drinking? *(1 mark)*
     Do you have to drink more than before to achieve
       intoxication or the desired effect? *(1 mark)*
  c Delirium tremens *(1 mark)*   /1

d i) 2 units *(1 mark)*   /3
    ii) 2 units *(1 mark)*
    iii) 1 unit *(1 mark)*
e Man – 21 units *(1 mark)*   /2
    Woman – 14 units *(1 mark)*

Summary

The treatment of alcohol abuse is initially through a detoxification regime, using chlordiazepoxide in a reducing dose. The patient also requires vitamin supplementation as they have not been eating properly prior to their admission. Referral to the psychiatry team can be of benefit so they are aware of the patient, however the patient should be informed of the effects of alcohol and strongly advised to stop drinking, and it should be left to the patient to refer themselves to the services following discharge, as this ensures they are willing to stop, and wish to have help.

6 a Acute pancreatitis *(1 mark)* due to alcohol *(1 mark)*   /2
  b *(1 mark for each correct answer, maximum 3 marks)*   /3
      Gall stones *(1 mark)*
      Trauma *(1 mark)*
      Steroids *(1 mark)*
      Mumps *(1 mark)*
      Autoimmune *(1 mark)*
      Scorpion bite *(1 mark)*
      Hyperlipidaemia *(1 mark)*
      ERCP *(1 mark)*
      Drugs *(1 mark)*
  c He is in withdrawal from alcohol, and has delirium   /1
      tremens *(1 mark)*
  d *(1 mark for each correct answer, maximum 3 marks)*   /3
      Confusion *(1 mark)*
      Disorientation *(1 mark)*
      Agitation *(1 mark)*
      Tremors *(1 mark)*
      Anxiety *(1 mark)*
      Seizures *(1 mark)*
  e Chlordiazepoxide *(1 mark)*   /1

Summary

Delirium tremens commonly occurs 2 days after a patient has been admitted, and they become acutely confused, often with visual or auditory hallucinations. There may be physical manifestations of their withdrawal, such as tremors, nausea and vomiting.

7 a *(1 mark for each correct answer, maximum 3 marks)* `/3`

A refusal to maintain body weight at or above a
   minimally normal weight for age and height
   (1 mark) (usually less than 85% of ideal
   body weight, or BMI less than 17.5)

Intense fear of gaining weight or becoming fat *(1 mark)*

Disturbance in the way one's body weight or
   shape is experienced, with denial of current
   low body weight *(1 mark)*

Amenorrhoea in postmenarcheal females of
   at least three menstrual cycles *(1 mark)*

b *(1 mark for each correct answer, maximum 3 marks)* `/3`

Purging activities *(1 mark)*

Vomiting *(1 mark)*

Laxative abuse *(1 mark)*

Diuretic use *(1 mark)*

Excessive exercise *(1 mark)*

c Weight/height × height = 44/1.6 × 1.6 = 17.2 *(1 mark)* `/1`

d *(1 mark for each correct answer, maximum 4 marks)* `/4`

Hypotension *(1 mark)*

Muscle atrophy *(1 mark)*

Dental cavities *(1 mark)*

Depression *(1 mark)*

Electrolyte disturbances *(1 mark)*

Kidney stones *(1 mark)*

Constipation *(1 mark)*

Summary

Anorexia presents with a body weight more than 25% below standard, an intense wish to be thin, amenorrhoea, distorted body image, and fear of being fat. The patient eats very little, and may purge by inducing vomiting, or takes excessive exercise. Psychological treatment may be necessary, through family therapy, social support, cognitive therapy to change the patient's attitude towards eating, and behavioural therapy with strict regimes.

Bulimia is characterised by episodes of uncontrollable eating followed by compensation such as vomiting, laxative abuse, or excess exercise. They may present with cardiac arrhythmias, renal damage, urinary infections, pitted teeth, epilepsy, tetany and weakness. Management is with antidepressants and group therapy.

8 a *(1 mark for each correct answer, maximum 2 marks)* `/2`

Obsessive compulsive disorder *(1 mark)*

Agoraphobia *(1 mark)*

Generalised anxiety disorder *(1 mark)*
b *(1 mark for each correct answer, maximum 4 marks)*   /4
Dyspnoea *(1 mark)*
Chest pain *(1 mark)*
Dysphagia *(1 mark)*
Nausea *(1 mark)*
Tremor *(1 mark)*
Indigestion *(1 mark)*
Sexual dysfunction *(1 mark)*
Dry mouth *(1 mark)*
Headache *(1 mark)*
c *(1 mark for each correct answer, maximum 2 marks)*   /2
Antidepressants (SSRIs) *(1 mark)*
Anxiolytics (benzodiazepines) *(1 mark)*
Beta-blockers *(1 mark)*
d Cognitive behavioural therapy *(1 mark)*   /2
Psychotherapy *(1 mark)*

Summary

Obsessive compulsive disorder is a condition in which the sufferer experiences recurrent intrusive thoughts regarding a fear or impulsive, which is usually accompanied by a feeling of anxiety. This is often relieved somewhat by carrying out the action a certain way, or number of times, such as repeated hand washing. Agoraphobia is a fear of open spaces, which sufferers having anxiety on leaving the home.

9 a Dementia is a generalised impairment of intellect,   /3
memory and personality, without impairment of
consciousness *(1 mark)*
It is an acquired, usually irreversible disorder,
typically occurring after the age of 65 *(1 mark)*
The symptoms should have been present for
more than 6 months *(1 mark)*
b Alzheimer's *(1 mark)*   /3
Vascular *(1 mark)*
Lewy body *(1 mark)*
c *(1 mark for each correct answer, maximum 2 marks)*   /2
Infection *(1 mark)*
Biochemical abnormalities *(1 mark)*
Endocrine *(1 mark)*
Cancer with brain metastases *(1 mark)*
d He may return home with a social package and   /2
respite care *(1 mark)*

He may require placement in a dementia
specialised home *(1 mark)*

Summary

There are several causes of dementia, such as Alzheimer's disease, vascular dementia, Lewy body dementia, Wernicke's encephalopathy, frontotemporal, Pick's disease, Huntington's chorea, CJD, hypothyroidism, diabetes, anoxia, space-occupying lesions, head trauma or infection. The incidence of dementia increases with age, with 1% of under 65s affected, 6% of 75–79-year-olds, and 45% of those over 95 affected.

10 a 23/30 *(1 mark)*　　　　　　　　　　　　　　　　　　 /1

  b Widening of the sulci *(1 mark)*　　　　　　　　　　　 /2
    Enlargement of the ventricles *(1 mark)*

  c *(1 mark for each correct answer, maximum 4 marks)*　 /4
    FBC – WCC can show chronic infections, RBCs can
      alter due to vitamin deficiencies *(1 mark)*
    U+E – electrolyte abnormalities can cause
      confusion *(1 mark)*
    TFT – hypothyroidism can cause
      pseudodementia *(1 mark)*
    CRP and ESR – any autoimmune disease *(1 mark)*
    Calcium – malignant syndrome *(1 mark)*
    Vitamin B12 and folate – Wernicke's
      encephalopathy *(1 mark)*

  d *(1 mark for each correct answer, maximum 2 marks)*　 /2
    Treatment may be given when the MMSE is
      between 10–20/30. *(1 mark)*
    Cholinesterase inhibitors (rivastigmine) *(1 mark)*
    NMDA receptor antagonists (memantine) *(1 mark)*

  e Exclude any reversible cause of dementia *(1 mark)*　 /3
    Assess psychological and social aspects – patient may
      wish to write a will whilst they can, or decide
      about lasting power of attorney *(1 mark)*
    Discuss the options for care at home, respite
      care, and residential homes *(1 mark)*

Summary

The first step in treating dementia is to exclude any reversible cause of the dementia, in order to prevent further deterioration. This is done with a thorough physical examination, and the above investigations.

In the long term, the psychological and social issues should be assessed, and provided for. The patient may wish to write a will, or decide about lasting power of attorney, whilst they still have the capacity to do so.

Patients should be treated at home wherever possible to limit confusion, possibly with house adaptations, social workers, and day care to assist both the patient and family. Respite care should also be offered to allow the carer a break, or a permanent residential home may be required. Hospital care is usually provided when extensive nursing care is needed, or the patient can no longer cope in the community, becoming unwell.

11 a Delirium is an acute *(1 mark)* reversible condition   `/3`
(1 mark) characterised by an impairment of
consciousness due to a physical illness *(1 mark)*

  b *(1 mark for each correct answer, maximum 3 marks)*   `/3`
Infection *(1 mark)*
Fever *(1 mark)*
Drug or alcohol intoxication or withdrawal *(1 mark)*
Organ failure *(1 mark)*

  c *(1 mark for each correct answer, maximum 4 marks)*   `/4`
Delirium is acute onset, dementia is insidious *(1 mark)*
Delirium follows a fluctuating course, dementia is
   stable or progressive if vascular *(1 mark)*
Delirium has impaired consciousness, dementia
   has normal consciousness *(1 mark)*
Delirious patients have disorganised thinking, dementia
   patients have impoverished thinking *(1 mark)*
Perceptual disturbance is common in delirium,
   not in dementia *(1 mark)*
In delirium alertness is usually impaired, dementia
   patients are alert *(1 mark)*

  d *(1 mark for each correct answer, maximum 3 marks)*   `/3`
Meals on wheels *(1 mark)*
Cleaner *(1 mark)*
Assistance with washing and dressing *(1 mark)*
Help with shopping *(1 mark)*

Summary

If a patient is admitted with acute confusion they should always be screened for infection and be deemed medically fit before referral to the psychiatry team. Delirium is very common in elderly patients with minor infections, and drug intoxication or withdrawal may also cause confusion. These things must be ruled out before a diagnosis of dementia can be made.

14 Paediatrics

QUESTIONS

1 Timothy, a 4-month-old baby, is brought in by his mother who is feeling quite anxious. She tells you that he has had a cold for a few days with persistent coughing and wheezing but that he has now become breathless and drowsy. On examination you observe respiratory distress, expiratory wheeze and fine end inspiratory crackles.

   a Give two signs of respiratory distress in a child.   *2 marks*

   b What is the likely diagnosis and its causative agent?   *2 marks*

   c Suggest two possible differential diagnoses.   *2 marks*

   d Explain the pathophysiology of this disease.   *2 marks*

   e Give three investigations you would request.   *3 marks*

   f Outline your supportive management for this patient.   *2 marks*

2 You are following up the progress of Alice, a 3-year-old girl in your outpatients clinic. You learn that she is taking longer than her peers in reaching her milestones and is attending a special nursery. As a baby she was delivered preterm, developed early hand preference and abnormalities in tone and posture. Last week one of the physiotherapists assessed her contractures and range of movement.

   a What are the four categories in the developmental assessment and give an example of each.   *4 marks*

   b What is the diagnosis and how would you define it?   *2 marks*

   c Name two common associations of this disease.   *2 marks*

   d Suggest two possible causes of this condition.   *2 marks*

   e Name three members of the multidisciplinary team that may help with Alice's management.   *3 marks*

3 Ajay, a 3-year-old boy, is brought in by his father who feels he is constipated. He reports that his child only opens his bowels once every 4 days with dry hard pellets that are very painful to pass.

Complete SAQs for Medical Finals By P. Stather et al, Published 2010 by Blackwell Publishing, ISBN: 978-1-4501-8928-6.

   a Name three questions you would ask him
     about the constipation.   *3 marks*
   b Name two organic causes of constipation in the
     paediatric population.   *2 marks*
   c Name two management options available for
     functional constipation.   *2 marks*
   d Give three different types of medications
     available for the treatment of constipation in
     any age group.   *3 marks*

4 Clive, a 2-year-old boy, is rushed into A & E because his mother
is extremely worried. She explains that he developed a runny
nose yesterday but today he is having difficulty breathing and
you observe he has a stridor-like cough.
   a Other than croup, give two differential diagnoses.   *2 marks*
   b What is the medical name for croup, and
     what is the common pathogen causing it?   *2 marks*
   c What must you not do with this patient?   *1 mark*
   d On examining him he is tachypnoeic, tachycardic and
     cyanotic. Outline three aspects of your immediate
     management.   *3 marks*
   e What is the pathophysiology of the condition?   *2 marks*

5 James, a 12-year-old boy, suffers from cystic fibrosis and suffers from frequent chest infections requiring occasional hospital
admissions. He was diagnosed with cystic fibrosis after suffering
a meconium ileus and failing to thrive.
   a What is the mode of inheritance and the
     most common defective gene involved?   *2 marks*
   b Explain the pathophysiology of this condition.   *2 marks*
   c What organisms are likely to colonise his
     respiratory tract?   *2 marks*
   d Give three abnormalities you may observe on
     examining him.   *3 marks*
   e Name one investigation available for diagnosing
     cystic fibrosis.   *1 mark*

6 Imran is a 3-year-old boy with learning difficulties, who has good
social skills but is frequently admitted with chest infections. On
examining Imran you diagnose another chest infection, and hear
an audible heart murmur. You also notice he has widely spaced
eyes, and check his hands which reveal a single palmar crease.

a What is the diagnosis and explain its aetiology. *2 marks*
b Give two differential diagnoses for global
   developmental delay. *2 marks*
c Give four further signs identifiable on
   examination of patients with the condition
   identified in part (a). *4 marks*
d Give two conditions these children are
   more likely to develop later in life. *2 marks*

7 Paul is 5 years old and initially doing well in the early years but his mother is worried about him as he has started having difficulty walking and climbing the stairs. On examination you observe him and notice that when he stands up he puts his hands on his thighs and his calf muscles look particularly big. You suspect a genetic condition.
a What is the diagnosis and its mode of inheritance? *2 marks*
b Explain the pathophysiology of this condition. *2 marks*
c What three investigations will you request to
   prove your diagnosis? *3 marks*
d Give four of the multidisciplinary team's treatment
   options. *4 marks*
e Give two complications of this disease. *2 marks*

8 Maisha, a 4-year-old girl who recently moved to the UK from Nigeria with her parents, is rushed into A & E by her father. He states that she was previously well but suddenly over the last 4 hours became very unwell, feverish and is constantly drooling. On examination she is sitting in a characteristic posture, is tachycardic and a harsh inspiratory stridor is audible.
a What is the life-threatening diagnosis? *1 mark*
b What is the likely organism and explain why this
   condition is rare in the UK. *2 marks*
c Describe the macroscopic appearance of the
   epiglottis in this condition. *1 mark*
d Give four aspects of your immediate management. *4 marks*
e What is the major life-threatening
   complication of this disease? *1 mark*
f A blood gas was taken – what does it show? *1 mark*

pH	7.25	(7.35–7.45)
pO_2	15	(11–13)
pCO_2	5.4	(4.5–6)

Bicarb   16   (21–28)
BE   –6   (+/–2)

9 George, a 15-month-old baby boy, is brought in to see you because his mother reports that he has not gained any weight. His centiles worry you as he has dropped two centiles for his weight and you suspect failure to thrive.

  a Give four questions you would like to ask
     his mother.   *4 marks*
  b Define failure to thrive.   *1 mark*
  c If a child is on the tenth centile for height
     what does that mean?   *2 marks*
  d Give four causes of failure to thrive.   *4 marks*

10 Jake, a normally healthy 3 year old boy, is brought in by his father who says that Jake has been becoming gradually more unwell with a fever. Today Jake has a very high temperature, and seemed to be having some kind of fit, but it only lasted for a short time.

  a Give three questions you would like to
     ask about the fit.   *3 marks*
  b From the history, Jake had an isolated generalised
     tonic clonic seizure. What is the likely diagnosis? *1 mark*
  c Name three other causes of a seizure.   *3 marks*
  d His father is very worried: what reassurance
     will you give him, and how will you
     advise him to prevent further occurrences?   *4 marks*

11 Grace, a 7-year-old girl, is rushed in to see you by her mother who is very worried. She states that for the past few hours she has had a fever, headache, neck stiffness and light hypersensitivity. You examine her to find she is Kernig's sign positive and you notice a non-blanching purpuric rash on her abdomen.

  a What is the likely diagnosis?   *1 mark*
  b How do you elicit Kernig's sign?   *3 marks*
  c Name one of the likely organisms responsible. *1 mark*
  d Give three signs of raised intracranial pressure. *3 marks*
  e Give four investigations you will request.   *4 marks*
  f What two immediate treatments will you
     start for a patient with this diagnosis?   *2 marks*

12 Carl is a 1-week-old baby who is brought in by his mother who is quite distressed and tells you that he has turned slightly yellow.

a What four questions would you like to
ask his mother? *4 marks*

b After a few days his jaundice settles and
you attribute it to physiological jaundice.
Why does this occur in babies? *3 marks*

c The onset of jaundice is very important.
When is it more likely to be pathological? *2 marks*

d Give four pathological causes of jaundice. *4 marks*

13 Oliver, a 5-week-old baby boy, is brought in by his parents as
the health visitor is worried that he is failing to thrive. On further questioning you learn that he is projectile vomiting shortly
after feeds.

a What is the most likely diagnosis? *1 mark*

b Explain the pathophysiology of this condition. *2 marks*

c Describe the following ABG and explain
why it occurs. *2 marks*

pH	7.47	(7.35–7.45)
pO_2	12.1	(11–13)
pCO_2	5.2	(4.5–6)
Bicarb	33	(21–28)
BE	+8	(+/−2)

d How would you manage this patient in the short
and long term? *2 marks*

e A child is brought in clinically dehydrated and
admission weight is 22 kg. Calculate their
maintenance fluid requirements per hour, and
show your workings. *3 marks*

f Give four signs of severe dehydration in a baby. *4 marks*

14 You are the paediatric doctor who has just attended and are
called to attend a difficult delivery of a baby thought to be in
distress due to an abnormal CTG tracing. On your arrival the
full-term baby has a heart rate of 120, is crying normally, has
good muscle flexion and is pink.

a Define full term. *1 mark*

b Name four high-risk situations during delivery
where a paediatrician needs to be called. *4 marks*

c Name five parts of a neonatal examination. *5 marks*

Paediatrics

ANSWERS

1 a *(1 mark for each correct answer, maximum 2 marks)*   **/2**
Tachypnoea *(1 mark)*
Subcostal, intercostal and sternal recession *(1 mark)*
Nasal flaring *(1 mark)*
Use of abdominal muscles *(1 mark)*
Tracheal tug *(1 mark)*

b Bronchiolitis *(1 mark)*   **/2**
RSV (respiratory syncytial virus) *(1 mark)*

c *(1 mark for each correct answer, maximum 2 marks)*   **/2**
Pneumonia *(1 mark)*
Viral wheeze *(1 mark)*
Meningitis *(1 mark)*

d *(1 mark for each correct answer, maximum 2 marks)*   **/2**
Bronchioles become inflamed *(1 mark)*
Secrete mucus *(1 mark)*
Oedema and necrosis cause obstruction of the
  airways *(1 mark)*

e *(1 mark for each correct answer, maximum 3 marks)*   **/3**
Bloods – FBC, CRP, U+E *(1 mark each, maximum 2 marks)*
Chest x-ray *(1 mark)*
Nasopharyngeal aspirate *(1 mark)*

f *(1 mark for each correct answer, maximum 2 marks)*   **/2**
Oxygen via a headbox *(1 mark)*
Respiratory support *(1 mark)*
Fluid and nutritional support *(1 mark)*

Summary
Patients present following a cold with increasing difficulty breathing and poor feeding. Bronchiolitis is a self-limiting viral infection which causes small airway obstruction and tends to affect those under 18 months. A chest x-ray may show hyperinflated lungs and a nasopharyngeal aspirate can be used to identify the virus from respiratory secretions.

2 a Gross motor skills, e.g. sitting, walking, running `/4`
(1 mark)
Fine motor skills, e.g. hand use, pincer grip,
throwing, drawing *(1 mark)*
Speech and language skills, e.g. speaking words,
understanding, role play *(1 mark)*
Social skills, e.g. social play, eating, toilet trained
(1 mark)

b Cerebral palsy *(1 mark)* `/2`
It is an irreversible, non-progressive insult to a
young child's brain, typically affecting movement
and posture *(1 mark)*

c *(1 mark for each correct answer, maximum 2 marks)* `/2`
Epilepsy *(1 mark)*
Learning difficulties *(1 mark)*
Hearing and visual loss *(1 mark)*
Incontinence *(1 mark)*

d *(1 mark for each correct answer, maximum 2 marks)* `/2`
During pregnancy – infections (TORCH) *(1 mark)*
During delivery – hypoxic ischaemic encephalopathy,
traumatic birth/delivery *(1 mark)*
Early years – meningitis, head injury, encephalitis
(1 mark)

e *(1 mark for each correct answer, maximum 3 marks)* `/3`
Physiotherapy *(1 mark)*
Occupational therapy *(1 mark)*
Play therapist *(1 mark)*
Special needs school teacher *(1 mark)*
Dietician *(1 mark)*
SALT *(1 mark)*
Surgeons *(1 mark)*
Genetic counselling *(1 mark)*

Summary

In cerebral palsy the brain insult is not progressive but as the child grows and develops the clinical picture tends to change. There are different types of cerebral palsy such as athetoid, spastic, ataxic and mixed, which reflect the different areas of the brain damaged. Most children with the condition have multiple problems and a multidisciplinary team approach is required to address their varying needs.

3 a *(1 mark for each correct answer, maximum 3 marks)* `/3`
Dietary history including fluid intake *(1 mark)*
Abdominal symptoms such as pain, bloating,
  nausea *(1 mark)*
Social history and setting *(1 mark)*
How did it start/constipation onset – was it
  present at birth? *(1 mark)*
Was the passage of meconium delayed? *(1 mark)*

b *(1 mark for each correct answer, maximum 2 marks)* `/2`
Hirschsprung's disease *(1 mark)*
Stenotic lesions *(1 mark)*
Anal pain due to fissures *(1 mark)*
Neuromuscular disease *(1 mark)*
Hypothyroidism *(1 mark)*

c *(1 mark for each correct answer, maximum 2 marks)* `/2`
Dietary changes to increase fibre, increase fluids,
  encourage exercise *(1 mark)*
Laxative/faecal softeners *(1 mark)*
Anaesthetic gel to relieve pain of anal fissures *(1 mark)*
Behavioural therapy (e.g. rewards) *(1 mark)*

d *(1 mark for each correct answer, maximum 3 marks)* `/3`
Bulking agents – Fybogel *(1 mark)*
Stimulant laxatives – senna *(1 mark)*
Stool softeners – arachis oil enema *(1 mark)*
Osmotic laxative – lactulose *(1 mark)*

Summary

As children have a wide range of bowel habits the diagnosis of constipation is assessed on stool hardness and pain on defecation rather than bowel frequency. Functional constipation is managed by bowel training, preventing relapses and regular follow-ups. It is also important to encourage good nutrition and encourage high-fibre food intake including bran, fruit, and vegetables.

4 a *(1 mark for each correct answer, maximum 2 marks)* `/2`
Acute epiglottitis *(1 mark)*
Foreign body *(1 mark)*
Anaphylaxis *(1 mark)*

b Acute laryngotracheobronchitis *(1 mark)* `/2`
Parainfluenza virus *(1 mark)*

c Do not examine the child's throat – this could `/1`
precipitate obstruction *(1 mark)*

d *(1 mark for each correct answer, maximum 3 marks)*   /3
Keep child calm *(1 mark)*
Inform a senior paediatrican and anaesthetist
   immediately *(1 mark)*
Nebulised adrenaline and oxygen *(1 mark)*
Steroids *(1 mark)*
Paediatric intensive care *(1 mark)*

e *(1 mark for each correct answer, maximum 2 marks)*   /2
Inflamed mucosa due to the virus causes increased
   secretions *(1 mark)*
Subglottic narrowing causes stridor *(1 mark)*
Children have a narrow trachea so even a small
   amount of inflammation is potentially
   dangerous *(1 mark)*

Summary

Patients with croup present with a classic barking cough. Croup usually affects children up to 2 years old and is very common in the win-
ter months. Most cases resolve spontaneously, however if obstruction is
likely then immediate intubation is vital in order to protect the fragile
airway. Due to the size of the trachea and upper airways in young children, a small decrease in the diameter is potentially life threatening.

5 a Autosomal recessive *(1 mark)*   /2
ΔF508 on chromosome 7q *(1 mark)*

b *(1 mark for each correct answer, maximum 2 marks)*   /2
Defective CFTR (cystic fibrosis transmembrane
   conductance regulator) *(1 mark)*
Decreased chloride transport *(1 mark)*
Thick viscous secretions prone to luminal
   obstruction *(1 mark)*

c *(1 mark for each correct answer, maximum 2 marks)*   /2
Staphylococcus aureus (1 mark)
Haemophilus influenzae (1 mark)
Pseudomonas (1 mark)

d *(1 mark for each correct answer, maximum 3 marks)*   /3
Malnutrition *(1 mark)*
Hyperinflated chest *(1 mark)*
Coarse crepitations at the lung bases *(1 mark)*
Expiratory rhonchi *(1 mark)*
Clubbing *(1 mark)*
Nasal polyps *(1 mark)*

  e *(maximum 1 mark)* **/1**
    Sweat test *(1 mark)*
    Antenatal tests – chorionic villus sampling *(1 mark)*
    Karyotyping *(1 mark)*

Summary

Patients with cystic fibrosis may present in the neonatal period with meconium ileus, or later in life with respiratory problems. Cystic fibrosis is a common disease with a population carrier rate of 1 in 25. The most common mutation involves the ΔF508 gene. This gene is responsible for chloride and sodium membrane transport in epithelial cells, so transport dysfunction results in thick viscous secretions in some organs including the respiratory and gastrointestinal systems. This causes increased susceptibility to respiratory infections, malabsorption and infertility.

6 a Down's syndrome *(1 mark)* **/2**
    Trisomy 21 – most commonly due to
      non-disjunction at meiosis *(1 mark)*

  b *(1 mark for each correct answer, maximum 2 marks)* **/2**
    Any chromosomal abnormality, e.g. Turner's
      syndrome, Klinefelter's syndrome *(1 mark)*
    Foetal alcohol syndrome *(1 mark)*
    Abuse and neglect *(1 mark)*
    Congenital hypothyroidism *(1 mark)*
    Trauma *(1 mark)*
    CNS malformation *(1 mark)*

  c *(1 mark for each correct answer, maximum 4 marks)* **/4**
    General – neonatal hypotonia *(1 mark)*
    Head – flat occiput *(1 mark)*
    Face – epicanthic folds *(1 mark)*, round face *(1 mark)*,
      upward-sloping palpebral fissures *(1 mark)*,
      protruding tongue *(1 mark)*
    Eyes – strabismus *(1 mark)*, nystagmus *(1 mark)*,
      Brushfield spots *(1 mark)*, cataracts *(1 mark)*
    Arms and legs – fifth finger clinodactyly *(1 mark)*,
      sandal gap *(1 mark)*

  d *(1 mark for each correct answer, maximum 2 marks)* **/2**
    Leukaemia *(1 mark)*
    Alzheimer's disease *(1 mark)*
    Pulmonary hypertension *(1 mark)*
    Premature aging *(1 mark)*
    Cataracts *(1 mark)*
    Conductive hearing loss *(1 mark)*

Summary

The most common form of congenital global developmental delay is Down's syndrome. The chromosomal abnormality present is chromosome 21 trisomy with the extra chromosome commonly being of maternal origin and the incidence increases with advancing maternal age. Children will have varying levels of learning disability and can often be introduced into mainstream schools. There is a wide range of signs for this condition, and investigations for cardiac defects should be performed.

7 a Duchenne muscular dystrophy *(1 mark)* /2
X-linked recessive *(1 mark)*

b *(1 mark for each correct answer, maximum 2 marks)* /2
Gene mutation on Xp21 *(1 mark)*
Dystrophin is absent which is important for muscle architecture *(1 mark)*
Muscle is lost and replaced by adipose cells *(1 mark)*

c *(1 mark for each correct answer, maximum 3 marks)* /3
Creatinine kinase *(1 mark)*
EMG *(1 mark)*
Muscle biopsy *(1 mark)*
Genetic tests *(1 mark)*

d *(1 mark for each correct answer, maximum 4 marks)* /4
Medical – steroids, treat cardiomyopathy *(1 mark)*
Surgery – correct contractures *(1 mark)*
Physiotherapy *(1 mark)*
Education *(1 mark)*
Counselling *(1 mark)*

e *(1 mark for each correct answer, maximum 2 marks)* /2
Limb contractures *(1 mark)*
Scoliosis *(1 mark)*
Cardiomyopathy *(1 mark)*
Respiratory infections *(1 mark)*

Summary

Duchenne muscular dystrophy is an X-linked recessive neuromuscular disease involving the absence of dystrophin. Patients present with deteriorating muscle function, so find it increasingly difficult to walk, stand and sit. Dystrophin is needed for cell membrane stability and its deficiency leads to reduced glycoprotein interactions within the cell membrane.

8 a Acute epiglottitis *(1 mark)* /1
  b *Haemophilus influenzae* B *(1 mark)* /2
    Rare as vaccine now introduced *(1 mark)*
  c *(maximum 1 mark)* /1
    Cherry red *(1 mark)*
    Swollen and inflamed *(1 mark)*
  d *(1 mark for each correct answer, maximum 4 marks)* /4
    Airway, Breathing, Circulation *(1 mark)*
    Anaesthetist to intubate urgently *(1 mark)*
    IV access and fluids *(1 mark)*
    Antibiotics *(1 mark)*
    Consult senior and consider transfer to
      paediatric intensive care *(1 mark)*
  e Acute airway obstruction *(1 mark)* /1
  f Metabolic acidosis due to secondary sepsis from /1
    bacterial infection *(1 mark)*

Summary

Acute epiglottis is a rare but life-threatening emergency caused by *Haemophilus influenzae* infection, which tends to affect older children. It is becoming rare due to immunisation with the Hib vaccine, which is being introduced to infants. The important aspect of management is to protect the airway and administer appropriate antibiotics, which should be done by an experienced senior doctor and anaesthetist.

9 a *(1 mark for each correct answer, maximum 4 marks)* /4
    Antenatal history *(1 mark)*
    Obstetric history *(1 mark)*
    Birth history and any complications *(1 mark)*
    Birth weight *(1 mark)*
    Nutritional history *(1 mark)*
    Social history and family situation *(1 mark)*
    Try to assess sensitively for any signs of
      possible neglect *(1 mark)*
    Ask about parental heights *(1 mark)*
  b When current weight or rate of weight gain is /1
    lower than that of children of the same age
    and sex *(1 mark)*
  c Out of 100 children 10% would be expected /2
    to be shorter than him and 90% would be
    expected to be taller than him *(1 mark)*, for
    children of the same age and sex *(1 mark)*

d *(1 mark for each correct answer, maximum 4 marks)*   **/4**
Nutrition: poor diet *(1 mark)*
Abuse and neglect *(1 mark)*
Problems with feeding – cerebral palsy *(1 mark)*
Unable to retain food – gastro-oesophageal
    reflux *(1 mark)*
Unable to absorb food – coeliac disease *(1 mark)*
Metabolic disease *(1 mark)*
Down's syndrome or other congenital syndromes *(1 mark)*
Ongoing illness *(1 mark)*

Summary
Failure to thrive represents a failure in growth, emotional and developmental progress and can be due to many causes. There is no specific criterion for failure to thrive but certain criteria can warrant referral to a paediatrician. These include weight below the 2nd centile, height below the 2nd centile and the crossing of two centiles for either height or weight. It is important to determine the cause of failure to thrive, so treatment can be started promptly.

10 a *(1 mark for each correct answer, maximum 3 marks)*   **/3**
Before fit – temperature *(1 mark)*
During fit – how long *(1 mark)*, shaking *(1 mark)*,
    tongue biting *(1 mark)*, limbs involved *(1 mark)*,
    incontinence *(1 mark)*
After fit – feeling drowsy and sleepy *(1 mark)*
Any previous fits? *(1 mark)*
b Febrile convulsion *(1 mark)*   **/1**
c *(1 mark for each correct answer, maximum 3 marks)*   **/3**
Epilepsy *(1 mark)*
Head injury *(1 mark)*
Metabolic disturbance *(1 mark)*
Infection *(1 mark)*
Raised intracranial pressure, e.g. tumour *(1 mark)*
Drugs *(1 mark)*
d *(1 mark for each correct answer, maximum 4 marks)*   **/4**
Not epilepsy *(1 mark)*
Very common in children *(1 mark)*
Due to high temperature *(1 mark)*
Give antipyretic to control temperature *(1 mark)*
Prevent injury by removing nearby objects,
    but don't restrict the child *(1 mark)*

Has a very good prognosis as they tend to
stop as the child grows *(1 mark)*
No increased risk of developing epilepsy *(1 mark)*

Summary

A febrile convulsion is a short-lived seizure occurring in young children typically under the age of 5 years and is caused by a fever. Young children have immature brains which are more susceptible to environmental stimulants and a fever is able to trigger a convulsion. It is important to give parents sufficient advice stating that the majority of children who have uncomplicated convulsions are at no greater risk than normal of developing epilepsy.

11 a Bacterial meningitis *(1 mark)*　　　　　　　　　　　/1
  b Seat patient upright *(1 mark)*　　　　　　　　　/3
    Flex hip and knees *(1 mark)*
    When you extend the knee it will be
      painful in the patient with meningitis *(1 mark)*
  c *(maximum 1 mark)*　　　　　　　　　　　　　　/1
    Neisseria meningitidis (1 mark)
    Streptococcus pneumoniae (1 mark)
    HiB *(1 mark)*
  d *(1 mark for each correct answer, maximum 3 marks)*　/3
    Papilloedema *(1 mark)*
    Reduced consciouness *(1 mark)*
    Neurological signs *(1 mark)*
    Cushing reflex *(1 mark)*
    Decerebrate posturing *(1 mark)*
  e *(1 mark for each correct answer, maximum 4 marks)*　/4
    Bloods – FBC, U+E, CRP *(1 mark each,*
      maximum 2 marks)
    ABG *(1 mark)*
    Blood culture *(1 mark)*
    Lumbar puncture if intracranial pressure not
      raised following CT *(1 mark)*
  f *(1 mark for each correct answer, maximum 2 marks)*　/2
    Third-generation cephalosporin *(1 mark)*
    Steroids to reduce inflammation *(1 mark)*
    IV fluids *(1 mark)*
    Analgesia *(1 mark)*
    Antipyretics *(1 mark)*
    Antibiotics for all close contacts *(1 mark)*

Summary

Meningitis is a common but very severe illness that can be either bacterial or viral. It is the result of organic invasion into the membranes surrounding the brain and spinal cord. Viral causes include mumps, Coxsackie virus and herpes virus. Patients present with fever, rash, neck stiffness and photophobia, possibly with reduced consciousness and neurological signs. The prognosis is dependant on early recognition and prompt treatment, but complications can include hydrocephalus, deafness, need for limb amputation and adrenal failure.

12 a *(1 mark for each correct answer, maximum 4 marks)*   ___/4___
   Onset of jaundice? *(1 mark)*
   Is the child unwell? *(1 mark)*
   Pale stools? *(1 mark)*
   Dark urine? *(1 mark)*
   Past medical history? *(1 mark)*
   Breast feeding? *(1 mark)*
   Pre-term? *(1 mark)*
   Was a previous sibling jaundiced? *(1 mark)*
   Mother's blood group and rhesus status? *(1 mark)*
   Family history? *(1 mark)*
   Birth and delivery history? *(1 mark)*

b There is increased destruction of red blood cells   ___/3___
   as the foetal haemoglobin is broken down
   (1 mark). This releases bilirubin into the blood
   (1 mark), and the immature liver is unable to
   conjugate and excrete it rapidly enough
   (1 mark)

c Within 24 hours of delivery *(1 mark)*   ___/2___
   Jaundice after about 2 weeks *(1 mark)*

d *(1 mark for each correct answer, maximum
   4 marks)*   ___/4___
   Rhesus and ABO incompatibility *(1 mark)*
   Glucose-6-phosphate dehydrogenase
      (1 mark)
   Herditary spherocytosis *(1 mark)*
   Galactosaemia *(1 mark)*
   Gilbert's syndrome *(1 mark)*
   Bacterial infection *(1 mark)*
   Massive bruising *(1 mark)*
   Hypothyroid *(1 mark)*

Internal haemorrhage *(1 mark)*
Prematurity *(1 mark)*
Breast milk jaundice *(1 mark)*
Neonatal hepatitis *(1 mark)*
Cystic fibrosis *(1 mark)*
Biliary atresia *(1 mark)*

Summary

Neonatal jaundice is a very common presentation and is usually due to increased red blood cell breakdown, releasing bilirubin into the bloodstream, combined with a physiologically immature liver which is unable to clear it thus allowing bilirubin to accumulate. As the liver matures the condition is self-limiting. The many causes of neonatal jaundice are divided into conjugated and unconjugated.

13 a Pyloric stenosis *(1 mark)* ⬜ /1
  b Pylorus muscle becomes thickened due to ⬜ /2
    hypertrophy and hyperplasia *(1 mark)* causing
    gastric outlet obstruction *(1 mark)*
  c The ABG shows metabolic alkalosis *(1 mark)* ⬜ /2
    due to a high pH and high bicarbonate. This is
    due to frequent vomiting with loss of hydrogen
    and chloride ions which are secreted in the gastric
    secretions. Fluid loss will cause a raised $K+$ and
    hence hypochloraemic, hyperkalaemic metabolic
    alkalosis *(1 mark)*
  d Short term – give small meals more frequently ⬜ /2
      (1 mark)
    Long term – surgery – pyloromyotomy *(1 mark)*
  e *(1 mark for each correct answer, maximum 3 marks)* ⬜ /3
    100 ml per kg for the first 10 kg *(1 mark)*
    50 ml per kg for the second 10 kg *(1 mark)*
    20 ml per kg after this *(1 mark)*
    = 1540 ml/24 hr. Divide this by
      24 hrs = 64 ml per hour *(1 mark)*
  f *(1 mark for each correct answer, maximum 4 marks)* ⬜ /4
    Skin laxity *(1 mark)*
    Sunken eyes *(1 mark)*
    Sunken fontanelles *(1 mark)*
    Impaired peripheral circulation (increased capillary refill
      time to greater than 2 seconds) *(1 mark)*
    Lethargy *(1 mark)*

Summary

Pyloric stenosis is caused by pylorus muscle hypertrophy and hyperplasia developing in the first few weeks of life. Patients present with projectile vomiting directly after feeding, and are permanently hungry. There may be a palpable olive-sized mass in the epigastric region. Treatment is via surgical correction and division of the pylorus muscle.

14 a Infant born between 37 and 42 weeks' gestation   `/1`
(1 mark)

  b *(1 mark for each correct answer, maximum 4 marks)*   `/4`
Prematurity *(1 mark)*
Foetal distress *(1 mark)*
Meconium staining *(1 mark)*
Emergency caesarean *(1 mark)*
Abnormal foetus *(1 mark)*
PROM *(1 mark)*

  c *(1 mark for each correct answer, maximum 5 marks)*   `/5`
Skin – jaundice, cyanosis *(1 mark)*
Head – fontanelles *(1 mark)*
Eyes – cataract *(1 mark)*
Mouth – cleft lip *(1 mark)*
Chest – heart, lungs, murmurs *(1 mark)*
Abdomen – organomegaly *(1 mark)*
Limbs – talipes *(1 mark)*
Genitals – hypospadias, ambiguous genitalia
  (1 mark)
Hips – congenital dislocation of the hip *(1 mark)*
Back – midline defects *(1 mark)*
Face – dysmorphism *(1 mark)*

Summary

The APGAR score is a simple test which can be repeated quickly to assess the immediate health of a newborn baby after birth. The score is calculated using the heart rate, respiratory rate, muscle tone, reflex irritability and skin colour.

It is important that all babies are subject to a neonatal examination to identify any common abnormalities early, which can then be corrected.

15 Obstetrics

QUESTIONS

1 Eloise, a 17-year-old primigravida, is 30 weeks pregnant. She has just been to see her midwife at a routine antenatal appointment. Her BP is 160/95, her urine shows protein +++ and her ankles are very oedematous.

   a What is your diagnosis?   *1 mark*

   b Name three risk factors for developing
      this condition.   *3 marks*

   c Give two other symptoms this patient may have.   *2 marks*

   d Give four investigations you would order and
      state what abnormalities you would be
      looking for.   *4 marks*

   e Other than maternal or foetal death, name
      four serious complications which may occur
      in this patient.   *4 marks*

2 Maria is a 30-year-old woman who is 20 weeks pregnant with twins. She has had two previous uncomplicated pregnancies. Fortunately she and the babies are well and there have been no problems so far.

   a Give four problems associated with twin
      pregnancies.   *4 marks*

   b Apart from a multiple pregnancy, give four other
      indications for a caesarean section delivery.   *4 marks*

   c Name three complications to the mother from a
      caesarean delivery.   *3 marks*

   d How might twin pregnancies be classified?   *3 marks*

3 Marina, a 23-year-old primigravida, has her urine tested routinely by her midwife and it is shown to contain glucose. BMs were normal at her booking appointment. She does not have

Complete SAQs for Medical Finals By P. Stather et al, Published 2010 by
Blackwell Publishing, ISBN: 978-1-4501-8928-6.

a urinary tract infection and she is clinically well. You suspect gestational diabetes.

    a Give one thing you would do to confirm she has gestational diabetes.   *1 mark*

    b You receive confirmation that she has got gestational diabetes. Give two steps you would take to manage her conservatively.   *2 marks*

    c Give four problems that the foetus is more at risk of if the mother has diabetes.   *4 marks*

    d Give two complications that the foetus is at greater risk of in utero.   *2 marks*

    e Marina is unable to control her BMs with diet. Give two steps you might take next in her management.   *2 marks*

    f Give three risk factors for developing gestational diabetes.   *3 marks*

4 Roisin, a 25-year-old primigravida comes into A & E with continuous vomiting which has been going on for the past 12 hours. She thinks she is 8 weeks pregnant but has not been to see her GP yet to have her pregnancy confirmed. You suspect hyperemesis gravidarum.

    a On questioning she has abdominal pain and no urinary or bowel symptoms. Give four steps in your initial management.   *4 marks*

    b Her pregnancy test is positive and her vomiting settles with your treatment. You diagnose hyperemesis gravidarum. Give three conditions which are suggested by the presence of hyperemesis gravidarum.   *3 marks*

    c What two physical signs would concern you in this patient?   *2 marks*

    d As she has not eaten anything for 24 hours what would you expect to find on urine dip-testing?   *1 mark*

5 Tiffany, a 33-year-old primigravida, is at 38 weeks' gestation when she goes into labour spontaneously. Her membranes have ruptured and she has now been in labour for 6 hours. The midwife does a vaginal examination (VE) and notes that the patient is 2 cm dilated.

    a Give three features which are assessed during a VE in labour.   *3 marks*

b After 6 hours you would hope her cervix had
dilated by greater than 2 cm. Give two possible
explanations for this slow progress. *2 marks*

c Her last contraction was 30 minutes ago. She is
very distressed and in a lot of pain. What would
your next two steps be with regard to care of
the mother? *2 marks*

d Give three of the features that you are looking for
on the CTG that might indicate foetal distress. *3 marks*

e How long after delivery should the placenta be
expelled? *1 mark*

6 Catherine is a 30-year-old primigravida, who comes to you concerned about giving birth. She is worried about being in pain for
a long time but doesn't want to take painkillers as she has heard
that it might harm the baby.

a Give three different options for pain relief in
labour other than epidural and spinal anaesthetic. *3 marks*

b Give three maternal complications associated
with an epidural. *3 marks*

c What is the difference between an epidural and
a spinal anaesthetic? *2 marks*

d Give three contraindications to an epidural. *3 marks*

7 Beth, a 36-year-old multigravida, comes for her 20-week
ultrasound scan, and placenta praevia is diagnosed. She is
asymptomatic.

a Define placenta praevia. *1 mark*

b What are the three categories of placenta praevia? *3 marks*

c Name two risk factors for having placenta praevia. *2 marks*

d Once the patient reaches 36 weeks' gestation,
what two things would you do? *2 marks*

e Beth collapses whilst an inpatient and suffers a
significant vaginal bleed. Give four steps you
will take in order to save her life. *4 marks*

8 A routine HIV test is done on a 20-year-old Nigerian girl called
Monica on her initial consultation with her GP since she found
out she is pregnant. She is coming to see you today for the
result, which is positive.

a Give three steps you can take to offer Monica
support. *3 marks*

b Suggest two long-term provisions you can make
for her. *2 marks*

c She is concerned that the baby will be HIV
positive. Give two measures you can take to
prevent this. *2 marks*

d Give three other questions you would ask her. *3 marks*

e Apart from a repeat HIV test, what two other
tests would you like to perform? *2 marks*

f Apart from pregnancy give one other indication
for starting HAART therapy. *1 mark*

9 A 34-year-old woman called Myfanwy is brought into A & E
with vaginal bleeding and abdominal pain. She tells you that
she is currently 22 weeks pregnant and that she has had three
miscarriages in the past; none of which have involved trauma.

a What is the definition of a miscarriage? *1 mark*

b Other than PCOS give three causes of recurrent
miscarriage. *3 marks*

c Give three blood tests you would do when she
comes to a follow-up clinic appointment to look
for a cause for her miscarriages. *3 marks*

d Apart from these blood tests you arrange three
further investigations. What are these, and what
may they show? *3 marks*

e It is found that she has PCOS and is treated.
In 12 months' time, after treatment, she comes
to see you before attempting conception again.
State four other pieces of general pre-pregnancy
advice you would give. *4 marks*

10 Shelly is a 29-year-old multiparous woman who goes into
labour at 32 weeks. She comes into the delivery suite with
contractions coming strongly every 4 minutes. She has had two
previous healthy natural deliveries and has no current medical
problems herself.

a Before how many weeks' gestation is a labour
considered to be premature? *1 mark*

b Name three risk factors for premature labour. *3 marks*

c You attach a CTG monitor and hear that the baby's
heart rate is fine at 140 bpm and is not showing
any distress. You consider giving the mother
steroids to improve the infant's lung function

should delivery happen soon. Between how many
weeks' gestation are steroids justified to be given? *1 mark*

d Name one drug that can be used to postpone the
onset of labour. *1 mark*

e Shelly's waters break. You suspect she has a
group B *Streptococcus* infection. How do you
treat it? *1 mark*

f If untreated, give three problems
group B *Streptococcus* infection can potentially
cause in the neonate. *3 marks*

Obstetrics

ANSWERS

1 a Pre-eclampsia *(1 mark)* /1

  b *(1 mark for each correct answer, maximum 3 marks)* /3
    Family history of pre-eclampsia *(1 mark)*
    Being a primigravida *(1 mark)*
    Patient's past history of pre-eclampsia *(1 mark)*
    Multiple pregnancy *(1 mark)*
    With pre-existing hypertension, diabetes,
      autoimmune disorder, disorders with increased
      blood clotting *(1 mark)*
    Extremes of maternal age *(1 mark)*

  c *(1 mark for each correct answer, maximum 2 marks)* /2
    Headache *(1 mark)*
    Visual disturbance *(1 mark)*
    Abdominal pain *(1 mark)*

  d *(1 mark for each correct answer, maximum 4 marks)* /4
    FBC – thrombocytopenia *(1 mark)*
    Blood film – haemolysis *(1 mark)*
    Renal function – raised urea and creatinine *(1 mark)*
    Uric acid – elevated *(1 mark)*
    LFTs – reduced albumin, deranged liver enzymes
      (1 mark)
    24-hour urinary protein – >0.5 g in 24 hours *(1 mark)*
    Ultrasound – to detect IUGR and oligohydramnios
      (1 mark)
    Doppler to record placental blood flow. Will be
      reduced *(1 mark)*

  e *(1 mark for each correct answer, maximum 4 marks)* /4
    DIC *(1 mark)*
    Cerebral haemorrhage *(1 mark)*
    Acute renal failure *(1 mark)*
    Acute cardiac failure *(1 mark)*
    Pulmonary oedema *(1 mark)*
    Hepatic failure *(1 mark)*

HELLP syndrome *(1 mark)*
Seizures *(1 mark)*
Premature birth *(1 mark)*

Summary

Pre-eclampsia is defined as hypertension, proteinuria and oedema, and patients may also complain of headache, visual disturbance and abdominal pain. Patients presenting to antenatal clinic with high blood pressure should be regularly monitored for these signs, and symptoms, as this condition may progress rapidly to eclampsia, when the baby must be delivered.

2 a Twin–twin transfusion *(1 mark)*　　　　　　　　　　　`/4`
Increased risk of structural abnormalities *(1 mark)*
Malpresentation *(1 mark)*
Polyhydramnios *(1 mark)*
Locked twins *(1 mark)*
Conjoined twins *(1 mark)*
Low birth weight *(1 mark)*
Perinatal death *(1 mark)*
IUGR *(1 mark)*

b *(1 mark for each correct answer, maximum 4 marks)*　　　`/4`
More than one previous caesarean *(1 mark)*
Foetal distress *(1 mark)*
Malpresentation of foetus *(1 mark)*
Failed instrumental delivery *(1 mark)*
Foetal macrosomia *(1 mark)*
Severe pre-eclampsia *(1 mark)*
High gravida *(1 mark)*
Failed induction – prolonged labour *(1 mark)*
Placenta praevia *(1 mark)*
Obstructed labour *(1 mark)*
Cervical dystocia *(1 mark)*
IUGR and placental failure *(1 mark)*
Prolapse cord *(1 mark)*
Cephalo-pelvic disproportion *(1 mark)*
Maternal choice *(1 mark)*

c *(1 mark for each correct answer, maximum 3 marks)*　　　`/3`
Haemorrhage *(1 mark)*
Infection *(1 mark)*
Bladder/bowel injury *(1 mark)*
Thromboembolic disease *(1 mark)*

Risk of scar rupture in future pregnancies *(1 mark)*
Increased risk of future placenta praevia *(1 mark)*
d Monochorionic diamniotic *(1 mark)*   /3
Monochorionic monoamniotic *(1 mark)*
Dichorionic diamniotic *(1 mark)*

Summary

Every complication that may be found in a singleton pregnancy is found in increased frequency in multiple pregnancies. The commonest cause for a large-for-dates uterus is multiple pregnancy, but other important causes such as polyhydramnios should not be ignored. In monochorionic, monoamniotic pregnancies there is an increased risk of twin–twin transfusion syndrome and as such women with these pregnancies are monitored more frequently.

3 a Glucose tolerance test *(1 mark)*   /1
  b *(1 mark for each correct answer, maximum 2 marks)*   /2
Referral to specialist diabetes antenatal clinic *(1 mark)*
Advise a low-sugar diet, giving her written
  information on what to eat, and dietician
  follow-up *(1 mark)*
Advise her to monitor and record her blood sugar,
  to be discussed at a follow-up appointment in
  2 weeks from now *(1 mark)*
Explain the problems to the continuation of the
  pregnancy if her BMs are not well controlled
  (1 mark)
Encourage exercise *(1 mark)*
  c *(1 mark for each correct answer, maximum 4 marks)*   /4
Macrosomia *(1 mark)*
Shoulder dystocia *(1 mark)*
Respiratory distress syndrome *(1 mark)*
Neonatal jaundice *(1 mark)*
Polycythaemia *(1 mark)*
Hypoglycaemia *(1 mark)*
Obstructed labour *(1 mark)*
  d *(1 mark for each correct answer, maximum 2 marks)*   /2
Intrauterine death *(1 mark)*
Miscarriage *(1 mark)*
Hypoxia *(1 mark)*
Congenital abnormality (especially cardiac) *(1 mark)*
Organomegaly *(1 mark)*

e *(1 mark for each correct answer, maximum 2 marks)* ☐ /2

Initiate and educate regarding the start of an insulin
regime based on her BM readings *(1 mark)*

Ultrasound scan to check foetal health and size
(1 mark)

Arrange a date for elective caesarean, to avoid an
obstructed labour *(1 mark)*

f *(1 mark for each correct answer, maximum 3 marks)* ☐ /3

Maternal age of over 25 years *(1 mark)*

Race – Asian, Hispanic *(1 mark)*

Maternal obesity *(1 mark)*

Family history of type 2 diabetes *(1 mark)*

Previous personal history of an unexplained stillbirth
or delivery of a child over 4.5 kg in weight *(1 mark)*

Summary

All types of diabetes carry greater risks for the safety of a pregnancy. Glucose is able to cross the placenta thus increasing the supplies to the foetus, but insulin does not cross the placental barrier, thus leading to hyperglycaemia in the foetus if there is maternal hyperglycaemia. The foetus compensates by overproducing insulin which leads to hypoglycaemia after birth. Mothers with diabetes are offered extra support throughout their pregnancy and increased monitoring.

Women who have had gestational diabetes are more likely to get type 2 diabetes, and will require a postnatal glucose tolerance test, as well as advice to stay thin and physically active.

4 a *(1 mark for each correct answer, maximum 4 marks)* ☐ /4

Confirm pregnancy with blood and urine tests
(1 mark)

Dip urine for signs of infection *(1 mark)*

Admit patient *(1 mark)*

Cannulate *(1 mark)*

NBM *(1 mark)*

Take blood for FBC, CRP, U+E, TFTs, LFTs
(maximum 1 mark)

Rehydrate with normal saline *(1 mark)*

Give prochlorperazine (anti-emetic) *(1 mark)*

b *(1 mark for each correct answer, maximum 3 marks)* ☐ /3

Multiple pregnancy *(1 mark)*

Thyrotoxicosis in pregnancy *(1 mark)*

UTI in pregnancy *(1 mark)*
Molar pregnancy *(1 mark)*
c Tachycardia *(1 mark)* ___/2___
Hypotension *(1 mark)*
d Ketones *(1 mark)* ___/1___

Summary

Morning sickness in pregnancy is very common until the second trimester. Hyperemesis gravidarum is persistent vomiting in pregnancy which may result in large amounts of weight loss, dehydration and acidosis and can put both the mother's and the foetus's life in danger if not treated appropriately with IV fluids and electrolyte correction.

5 a *(1 mark for each correct answer, maximum 3 marks)* ___/3___
Consistency, effacement and dilatation of the cervix *(1 mark)*
Whether the membranes are intact *(1 mark)*
Colour of the amniotic fluid *(1 mark)*
Nature and presentation of the presenting part and its relationship to the ischial spines *(1 mark)*
Size of pelvic outlet *(1 mark)*
b Insufficient strength of uterine contractions *(1 mark)* ___/2___
Malpresentation of baby *(1 mark)*
Pelvic abnormality *(1 mark)*
c *(1 mark for each correct answer, maximum 2 marks)* ___/2___
Maternal observations *(1 mark)*
Start an infusion of oxytocin to speed up and increase the force of contractions *(1 mark)*
Ensure adequate pain relief and hydration for mother *(1 mark)*
Reassure mother and explain what is happening *(1 mark)*
d *(1 mark for each correct answer, maximum 3 marks)* ___/3___
Absence of accelerations *(1 mark)*
Presence of decelerations *(1 mark)*
Decreased baseline activity *(1 mark)*
Baseline tachycardia or bradycardia *(1 mark)*
e Within 30 minutes *(1 mark)* ___/1___

Summary

Labour is defined as the process by which the products of conception are expelled from the uterus after the 24th week of pregnancy.

There are three stages of labour. The first is dilatation, the second delivery of the baby and the third delivery of the placenta. If the placenta is not delivered within 30 minutes after the baby, then an injection of oxytocin is administered, possibly with surgical exploration if still not expelled. Normal labour in a primigravida can be up to 24 hours and 16 hours in a multigravida.

6 a *(1 mark for each correct answer, maximum 3 marks)* `/3`
Water immersion *(1 mark)*
TENS machine *(1 mark)*
Having a birth partner has been shown to reduce
    perception of pain *(1 mark)*
Pethidine injections *(1 mark)*
Entonox *(1 mark)*

b *(1 mark for each correct answer, maximum 3 marks)* `/3`
Epidural abscess *(1 mark)*
Hypotension *(1 mark)*
Urinary retention *(1 mark)*
Delayed second stage of labour due to decreased
    ability to push effectively *(1 mark)*
Nausea and vomiting *(1 mark)*
Headache *(1 mark)*
Inability to move freely *(1 mark)*
Increased chances of an instrumental delivery *(1 mark)*

c The difference is based on the anatomical location `/2`
    of where the anaesthetic is inserted *(1 mark)*
Epidural is inserted into the potential space that
    lies between the dura mater and the periosteum
    lining the inside of the vertebral canal *(1 mark)*
Spinal anaesthesia is induced by injecting
    small amounts of local anaesthetic into the
    cerebrospinal fluid (CSF) after having pierced
    the dura mater *(1 mark)*

d *(1 mark for each correct answer, maximum 3 marks)* `/3`
Abnormal bleeding *(1 mark)*
Skin infection at or near site *(1 mark)*
Hypovolaemia *(1 mark)*
Neurological disorders *(1 mark)*
Cardiovascular disease *(1 mark)*
Anatomical abnormalities of the vertebral column *(1 mark)*
Patient refusal *(1 mark)*
Lack of adequately trained staff *(1 mark)*

Summary

There are multiple techniques for controlling pain in labour, not all of which are pharmacological. Initial preparation of mothers during antenatal classes is vital as this increases their understanding and hence decreases their perception of pain. A calm, softly lit room is said to be soothing to women in labour and many women benefit from using alternative postures (e.g. exercise ball, birthing stool, birthing pool).

7 a When all or part of the placenta implants in the lower uterine segment and in front of the presenting part *(1 mark)*   /1

  b Lateral *(1 mark)*   /3
Marginal *(1 mark)*
Central *(1 mark)*

  c *(1 mark for each correct answer, maximum 2 marks)*   /2
Placenta praevia in previous pregnancy *(1 mark)*
Being multiparous *(1 mark)*
Previous caesarean *(1 mark)*

  d *(1 mark for each correct answer, maximum 2 marks)*   /2
Admit *(1 mark)*
Cross match *(1 mark)*
Elective caesarean *(1 mark)*

  e *(1 mark for each correct answer, maximum 4 marks)*   /4
ABC *(1 mark)*
Call for senior help immediately *(1 mark)*
Widebore IV access and fluids *(1 mark)*
Call blood bank for urgent blood (inform them of an obstetric emergency) *(1 mark)*
Take to theatre for urgent caesarean and possible hysterectomy *(1 mark)*

Summary

PV bleeds in pregnancy can be life threatening for both mother and baby. Abruptions can be revealed, concealed, and mixed, however all must be considered to contain a concealed component until this has been ruled out and the volume of blood loss is then known.

8 a *(1 mark for each correct answer, maximum 3 marks)*   /3
Make sure she has someone with her when she comes in for the result *(1 mark)*
Written information to take away with her *(1 mark)*
Follow-up appointment and counselling *(1 mark)*

Reassure her that her result will be confidential, but
request permission to inform the midwives who
will be working with her *(1 mark)*

b *(1 mark for each correct answer, maximum 2 marks)* ⬚ **/2**
Partner notification *(1 mark)*
Improving her sexual health, contraception *(1 mark)*
Lifestyle balance/keeping well *(1 mark)*
Refer patient to specialist *(1 mark)*

c *(1 mark for each correct answer, maximum 2 marks)* ⬚ **/2**
Elective caesarean delivery *(1 mark)*
Avoid breast feeding *(1 mark)*
Start mother on HAART regime antenatally at
28–32 weeks and give to the neonate for the
first 4–6 weeks of life *(1 mark)*

d *(1 mark for each correct answer, maximum 3 marks)* ⬚ **/3**
Does she or has she ever used illegal drugs? *(1 mark)*
Has she ever been raped? *(1 mark)*
Is her general health good? *(1 mark)*
Any weight loss, diarrhoea, fever, night sweats? *(1 mark)*
Number of sexual partners? *(1 mark)*

e *(1 mark for each correct answer, maximum 2 marks)* ⬚ **/2**
Hepatitis B and C *(1 mark)*
Viral load and CD4 count. *(1 mark)*
Other sexually transmitted infections – do triple
swabs if not done already as part of antenatal
testing *(1 mark)*

f *(maximum 1 mark)* ⬚ **/1**
Low or falling CD4 count *(1 mark)*
Post-exposure prophylaxis: occupational or sexual
(1 mark)

Summary

HIV tests are offered as part of routine antenatal testing to all
expectant mothers in Britain in order that a greater detection rate
will be achieved. The vertical transmission rate from mother to
baby is between 13% and 30% without treatment. Vertical transmission can be reduced by over 60% with the use of antiretrovi-
rals and reduced by 50% if babies are bottle fed. During labour it
is important that all care-givers are warned about the high-risk
status of the mother and that foetal scalp electrodes are avoided.

9 a The spontaneous expulsion of a foetus before ⬚ **/1**
24 weeks' gestation *(1 mark)*

b *(1 mark for each correct answer, maximum 3 marks)* /3

Hypothyroidism *(1 mark)*

Systemic lupus erythematosus *(1 mark)*

Protein C and S deficiency *(1 mark)*

Anti-phospholipid syndrome *(1 mark)*

Malformation of the uterus *(1 mark)*

Balanced translocation in either mother or father
(1 mark)

Fibroids *(1 mark)*

Asherman's syndrome *(1 mark)*

c *(1 mark for each correct answer, maximum 3 marks)* /3

FSH *(1 mark)*

LH *(1 mark)*

TFT *(1 mark)*

Prolactin *(1 mark)*

Sex hormone binding globulin *(1 mark)*

Testosterone *(1 mark)*

Protein C and S *(1 mark)*

Coagulation studies *(1 mark)*

d *(1 mark for each correct answer, maximum 3 marks)* /3

US scan to detect mucous fibroids or PCOS *(1 mark)*

Hysteroscopy can detect a malformation of uterus
(1 mark)

Karyotype – a balanced translocation may be found
(1 mark)

e *(1 mark for each correct answer, maximum 4 marks)* /4

Best time to travel is less than 24 weeks' gestation
(1 mark)

Take folic acid for 3 months prior to conception and
during pregnancy *(1 mark)*

Advise on smoking cessation and avoidance of alcohol *(1 mark)*

Not to eat any unpasteurised cheeses or pates – to
decrease the chances of listeriosis *(1 mark)*

Avoid cats: risk of toxoplasmosis *(1 mark)*

Advise on use of medications in pregnancy, what is
and what is not safe to take *(1 mark)*

Optimise diabetic control if patient is diabetic *(1 mark)*

Summary

Recurrent spontaneous miscarriage is the loss of three or more foe-
tuses all of which were under 500 g in weight. Women who have
suffered the trauma of three miscarriages are often concerned they

will never have a successful pregnancy, but you can reassure them that they still have a 70% chance of a normal pregnancy with their next conception.

10 a Before 37 weeks is premature *(1 mark)* `/1`

  b *(1 mark for each correct answer, maximum 3 marks)* `/3`
  Low socio-economic status *(1 mark)*
  Extremes of maternal age *(1 mark)*
  Heavy stressful work *(1 mark)*
  Smoking *(1 mark)*
  Substance misuse *(1 mark)*
  Cervical incompetence *(1 mark)*
  PROM (associated with infection) *(1 mark)*
  Multiple pregnancy *(1 mark)*
  Uterine anomalies *(1 mark)*
  Antepartum haemorrhage *(1 mark)*
  Previous pre-term delivery *(1 mark)*
  Maternal febrile illness *(1 mark)*
  Genital tract infection, e.g. group B *Streptococcus*
    (1 mark)

  c 28–34 weeks *(1 mark)* `/1`

  d *(maximum 1 mark)* `/1`
  Beta agonists
  Calcium channel blockers *(1 mark)*
  Nitric oxide donors (GTN) *(1 mark)*

  e IV Benzyl penicillin provided she has no allergies `/1`
    (1 mark)

  f Chest infection *(1 mark)* `/3`
  Septicaemia *(1 mark)*
  Meningitis *(1 mark)*
  (all within 3 months of age)

Summary

Premature babies have a poor chance of survival which is directly related to gestational age. Babies who are born severely premature are more likely to have long-term disabilities including cerebral palsy, visual impairment and respiratory difficulties. If they are between 28 and 34 weeks' gestation then steroids should be administered prior to delivery, and the paediatric team should be present at the birth.

16 Gynaecology

QUESTIONS

1 A couple come to see you in the clinic. Jill is 36 years old and Mark is 42. They have been having regular, unprotected sexual intercourse for 1 year with no success. Mark has two children from a previous relationship.

   a Give three questions you would ask Jill.   *3 marks*

   b Give three factors which could explain their failure to conceive, and a cause of each.   *3 marks*

   c Suggest three initial investigations.   *3 marks*

   d Jill's blood tests come back and everything is within normal ranges apart from her prolactin level which is 1500 IU/l. What is the likely diagnosis?   *1 mark*

   e Give two other symptoms Jill might be experiencing.   *2 marks*

   f Suggest one medical treatment you might prescribe.   *1 mark*

2 Vicki, a 25-year-old girl, is referred to you with lower abdominal pain. She has been admitted under the care of general surgeons and surgical causes have been excluded. They send her along to you (a gynaecologist) for your opinion, and after taking a thorough history you suspect PID.

   a Give two differential diagnoses.   *2 marks*

   b Other than abdominal pain, suggest four further symptoms Vicki may complain of.   *4 marks*

   c Give three causes of pelvic infection in the general population.   *3 marks*

   d Give two investigations you would perform on this patient.   *2 marks*

   e Your investigations confirm that Vicki has PID. Give three steps in Vicki's management.   *3 marks*

Complete SAQs for Medical Finals By P. Stather et al, Published 2010 by Blackwell Publishing, ISBN: 978-1-4501-8928-6.

3 Eileen, a 61-year-old lady, is referred to see you by her GP. Her main symptom is a blood-stained vaginal discharge, which has become heavier lately. She is otherwise well. On examination you find that she is obese with a BMI of 35 and a distended non-tender abdomen. Extensive investigations reveal a diagnosis of endometrial carcinoma.

a Suggest three differential diagnoses. *3 marks*

b Name three of the risk factors for endometrial cancer. *3 marks*

c Give three investigations you would order for a patient you suspect to have endometrial cancer. *3 marks*

d Histology reveals Eileen's cancer to be stage II. She requires a total abdominal hysterectomy and bilateral salpingo-oopherectomy. Other than haemorrhage, infection and the risks of general anaesthetic give three risks associated with this operation. *3 marks*

e Suggest two other gynaecological conditions which might require a hysterectomy. *2 marks*

4 A 35-year-old African lady comes to see you in clinic with menorrhagia. Her periods have become heavier over the past 5 years but increasingly so over the past year. She also reports feeling tired and lethargic all the time. She says she bleeds heavily for 10 days of the month, passing lots of clots, and has had to have time off work due to this. You suspect she has fibroids.

a Give three other possible causes of her menorrhagia. *3 marks*

b What three questions would you ask her to confirm or refute this? *3 marks*

c Suggest two investigations you would request to confirm the existence of a fibroid. *2 marks*

d It is found that she has a single large fibroid. Suggest two treatment options for this. *2 marks*

e Identify two of the risk factors for fibroids. *2 marks*

5 Gemma, a 30-year-old woman, presents to A & E complaining of lower abdominal pain. Her LMP was 8 weeks ago but her periods are usually irregular. She is currently sexually active. She has no change in bowel habit but 2 hours ago noticed some blood-stained vaginal discharge, and she has lost some more fresh blood since. She is in a lot of pain.

a Suggest three differential diagnoses. *3 marks*

b Give two biochemical investigations you
would request. *2 marks*

c Gemma's abdominal pain increases and
she also begins to complain of pain in
her shoulder. What is the most likely diagnosis? *1 mark*

d Her condition deteriorates. You decide to send
her to theatre urgently for a laparoscopy.
Give three things you would do to prepare
Gemma for theatre. *3 marks*

e Name three risk factors for this condition. *3 marks*

6 Jo, a 28-year-old woman, has been referred to gynaecology outpatients with pelvic pain that occurs before and during menstru-
ation and irregular uterine bleeding. She also reports post-coital
bleeding on occasion. Her periods have always been painful but
became worse over the past 2 years. You suspect endometriosis.

a Give two differential diagnoses for Jo's condition. *2 marks*

b Give three other gynaecological symptoms
you should ask Jo about. *3 marks*

c Suggest two features you might find on
examination of a woman with endometriosis. *2 marks*

d Nothing is found on examination. Jo says that
the pain is causing her serious disability with her
having to take a few days off work each month.
She is also feeling tired and lethargic. Give two
blood tests you would order, and why. *2 marks*

e Jo is scheduled for an exploratory laparoscopy.
Give one major complication specific to this
procedure. *1 mark*

7 Anne, a 54-year-old lady, comes to see you at your surgery. Her
periods have become irregular and heavier recently. On further
probing you find that she is often tearful and has been experiencing headaches lately. She asks you to open the window in
the surgery as she is feeling hot.

a Give two possible causes of her symptoms other
than menopause. *2 marks*

b Name two blood tests you would request. *2 marks*

c The tests show that Anne is perimenopausal
and she asks you about starting HRT. Give two
contraindications to starting her on HRT. *2 marks*

  d She also says that she is experiencing pain on
     intercourse and this is making her very unhappy
     as she used to enjoy an active sex life. Explain the
     pathophysiology behind this.   *1 mark*
  e Other than the symptoms mentioned above, give
     two further symptoms women may experience at
     menopause.   *2 marks*
  f There are two types of HRT, oestrogen only and
     oestrogen with progesterone. Which would you
     give to Anne and why? She has never had any
     abdominal or pelvic surgery.   *2 marks*

8 Agnes, a 65-year-old lady, comes to see you in clinic very embarrassed that she is starting to leak urine when she laughs or coughs. This has been a problem for the past 5 years but has worsened recently and she always wears a sanitary towel. She is concerned that she smells and it often puts her off going out with her friends.

  a What is the difference between stress and urge
     incontinence?   *2 marks*
  b Give three of the risk factors for developing
     stress incontinence.   *3 marks*
  c What might you find on vaginal examination
     in this patient?   *1 mark*
  d Suggest two conservative treatments you could
     offer Agnes.   *2 marks*
  e If conservative management fails, suggest
     one surgical method of intervention.   *1 mark*
  f How can the risk of uterine prolapse be avoided?
     Give two techniques.   *2 marks*

9 Anoushka, a 17-year-old girl, comes to your termination of pregnancy clinic. Her GP has done a pregnancy test which is positive. She thinks she is about 8 weeks pregnant. She wants a termination because she doesn't think she could cope with a baby and would not have the support of any family or a partner.

  a What investigation would you need to do before
     you can proceed?   *1 mark*
  b You confirm that she is 8 weeks pregnant
     and offer her a medical termination. Which
     two drugs are given?   *2 marks*
  c Name three contraindications to a medical
     termination.   *3 marks*

d Another patient called Catriona comes to the clinic requesting a termination. She is further on in her pregnancy and you offer her a surgical termination. Before you consent you outline to her some of the risks of the procedure. List three of these. *3 marks*

e Give three ways that complications after a termination can be minimised. *3 marks*

10 Angelina who is 23 years old is referred to you by her GP with oligomenorrhoea and menorrhagia. Her periods have always been erratic since menarche at 14 but more so since 16. You suspect she might have PCOS.

a Give three differential diagnoses apart from PCOS. *3 marks*

b What four further questions would you ask Angelina to differentiate between all of these options? *4 marks*

c Suggest three blood tests you would request and identify the abnormalities you would expect. *3 marks*

d Give two of the long-term sequalae of PCOS. *2 marks*

e Name two of the treatment options for PCOS. *2 marks*

Gynaecology
ANSWERS

1 a *(1 mark for each correct answer, maximum 3 marks)* /3
  Are her periods regular? *(1 mark)*
  Previous ectopics/miscarriages/terminations? *(1 mark)*
  Excess body hair? Acne? Weight gain? (PCOS)
    (1 mark)
  Dysmenorrhoea/menorrhagia? (thinking of
    endometriosis) *(1 mark)*
  History of STIs (thinking of PID) *(1 mark)*
  Is Jill taking any medication that could interfere
    with her ability to conceive? *(1 mark)*
b Failure to ovulate – excessive exercise, /3
    underweight, hyperprolactinaemia, PCOS,
    premature ovarian failure *(1 mark)*
  Fallopian tubes not patent – infection,
    endometriosis, adhesions *(1 mark)*
  Male: failure of sperm production – previous
    testicular radiotherapy, infection *(1 mark)*
c *(1 mark for each correct answer, maximum 3 marks)* /3
  Female:
  Measure blood levels of LH, FSH and oestradiol
    early in the follicular phase (days 2–6) *(1 mark)*
  Progesterone test – should be done mid-luteal phase
    (day 21 or 7 days before expected menses *(1 mark)*
  Measure blood levels of TSH, prolactin and
    testosterone if the woman's cycle is shortened,
    irregular or prolonged or if progesterone
    indicates anovulation *(1 mark)*
  Transvaginal USS if suspecting fibroids or PCOS
    (1 mark)
  Male:
  Semen sample for analysis should be taken after
    2–3 days' abstinence and repeated after 6 weeks
    if abnormal *(1 mark)*

d Pituitary adenoma *(1 mark)* /1

e *(1 mark for each correct answer, maximum 2 marks)* /2
Galactorrhoea *(1 mark)*
Menorrhagia *(1 mark)*
Bitemporal hemianopia *(1 mark)*
Diplopia *(1 mark)*

f Give a dopamine agonist, e.g. bromocriptine *(1 mark)* /1

Summary

Infertility is defined as failure to achieve conception after 12 months of regular unprotected sexual intercourse. Infertility can be due to male or female problems or a combination of both. Investigations should only be initiated after 12 months; before then couples should be offered advice and reassurance. Couples with fertility problems may be offered help in the form of IVF, GIFT or ZIFT. Other options include egg or sperm donation, surrogacy or adoption.

2 a *(1 mark for each correct answer, maximum 2 marks)* /2
Endometriosis *(1 mark)*
Ovarian cyst *(1 mark)*
Irritable bowel syndrome *(1 mark)*
Ectopic pregnancy *(1 mark)*

b *(1 mark for each correct answer, maximum 4 marks)* /4
Irregularity of menstrual cycle *(1 mark)*
Vaginal discharge *(1 mark)*
Dyspareunia *(1 mark)*
Urinary symptoms *(1 mark)*
Pain in relation to menstrual cycle *(1 mark)*
Pain in relation to eating *(1 mark)*
Any abdominal distension *(1 mark)*
Change to bowel habit *(1 mark)*
Blood in stools *(1 mark)*

c *(1 mark for each correct answer, maximum 3 marks)* /3
Post miscarriage *(1 mark)*
Post termination of pregnancy *(1 mark)*
Puerperal sepsis *(1 mark)*
Intrauterine contraceptive device *(1 mark)*

d *(1 mark for each correct answer, maximum 2 marks)* /2
Full STI screen – high vaginal, urethral and
endocervical swabs *(1 mark)*
Pregnancy test *(1 mark)*

Bloods – FBC, CRP *(maximum 1 mark)*
Transvaginal USS *(1 mark)*
Laparoscopy *(1 mark)*
e *(1 mark for each correct answer, maximum 3 marks)* `/3`
Analgesia *(1 mark)*
Antibiotics *(1 mark)*
Abstinence from intercourse for duration of
   treatment *(1 mark)*
Encourage partner notification and treatment
   (1 mark)
Patient education about safe sex *(1 mark)*
Follow-up according to results and local protocol
   (1 mark)

Summary

Triple swabs are often negative in patients who have PID because the infection is higher up within the genital tract. If left untreated, chronic pain can develop and the patient may be left infertile. Patients can be given the option of informing their partners themselves or, with their consent, this may be done anonymously by the genitourinary medicine clinic.

3 a *(1 mark for each correct answer, maximum 3 marks)* `/3`
Incomplete cessation of menses *(1 mark)*
Cervical cancer *(1 mark)*
Ovarian cancer *(1 mark)*
Cervical polyp *(1 mark)*
Endometrial polyp *(1 mark)*
Atropic vaginitis *(1 mark)*
  b *(1 mark for each correct answer, maximum 3 marks)* `/3`
Obesity *(1 mark)*
Long-term tamoxifen *(1 mark)*
Nulliparity *(1 mark)*
Late menopause *(1 mark)*
Diabetes *(1 mark)*
PCOS *(1 mark)*
Unopposed oestrogen stimulation *(1 mark)*
Age *(1 mark)*
  c *(1 mark for each correct answer, maximum 3 marks)* `/3`
Endometrial biopsy *(1 mark)*
Tumour marker (CA125) *(1 mark)*

Cervical smear *(1 mark)*
Pelvic USS *(1 mark)*
Hysteroscopy *(1 mark)*
Blood levels of FSH and LH *(1 mark)*
d *(1 mark for each correct answer, maximum 3 marks)* /3
Damage to urethra, ureters and bowel *(1 mark)*
Thromboembolism *(1 mark)*
Stress incontinence *(1 mark)*
Risk of herniation through scar site *(1 mark)*
e *(1 mark for each correct answer, maximum 2 marks)* /2
Severe endometriosis *(1 mark)*
Fibroids *(1 mark)*
Other gynaecological cancers *(1 mark)*
Menorrhagia, cause unknown *(1 mark)*
PID with chronic pain *(1 mark)*

Summary

Endometrial cancer typically presents with bleeding in postmenopausal women. Therefore, although many patients particularly on HRT, present with irregular bleeding, this diagnosis should be investigated. It may also occur in premenopausal women where it can be associated with irregular vaginal bleeding and menorrhagia. Diagnosis is by endometrial biopsy via a pipelle, and hysteroscopy to ensure no abnormalities are missed.

4 a *(1 mark for each correct answer, maximum 3 marks)* /3
Endometrial carcinoma (1 mark)
Adenomyosis *(1 mark)*
Inert or copper containing contraceptive device
  (1 mark)
Dysfunctional uterine bleeding *(1 mark)*
Endometriosis *(1 mark)*
Hypothyroidism *(1 mark)*
Clotting abnormalities *(1 mark)*
b *(1 mark for each correct answer, maximum 3 marks)* /3
History of recurrent miscarriage? *(1 mark)*
Increased urinary frequency? *(1 mark)*
Infertility? *(1 mark)*
Change in bowel habit? –constipation *(1 mark)*
Post-coital bleeding? *(1 mark)*
Dyspareunia? *(1 mark)*

c *(1 mark for each correct answer, maximum 2 marks)*   /2
Ultrasound of abdomen *(1 mark)*
Hysteroscopy *(1 mark)*
Laparoscopy. *(1 mark)*

d *(1 mark for each correct answer, maximum 2 marks)*   /2
Myomectomy *(1 mark)*
Uterine artery embolisation *(1 mark)*
Hysterectomy *(1 mark)*

e *(1 mark for each correct answer, maximum 2 marks)*   /2
Obesity *(1 mark)*
Race (African origin) *(1 mark)*
Family history *(1 mark)*
Age *(1 mark)*

Summary

Fibroids (also known as leiomyomas) are found in 20% of women of childbearing age. Women typically present with menorrhagia and symptoms of anaemia although in rarer cases they may complain of the pressure effects of large fibroids (such as bladder and bowel symptoms). Many women have several small fibroids which are asymptomatic, and treatment is therefore reserved for those where the fibroids are causing symptoms.

5 a *(1 mark for each correct answer, maximum 3 marks)*   /3
Ectopic pregnancy *(1 mark)*
Appendicitis *(1 mark)*
Rupture or haemorrhage of ovarian cyst *(1 mark)*
Miscarriage *(1 mark)*
Late period *(1 mark)*

b *(1 mark for each correct answer, maximum 2 marks)*   /2
Bloods – CRP, FBC, U+E, serum beta HCG
    (1 mark each)
Urinary pregnancy test *(1 mark)*

c Ruptured ectopic pregnancy *(1 mark)*   /1

d *(1 mark for each correct answer, maximum 3 marks)*   /3
2 large-bore cannulae in the antecubital fossa *(1 mark)*
IV fluids *(1 mark)*
Routine bloods – FBC, U+E, CRP, clotting, group
    and save *(maximum 1 mark)*
Keep NBM *(1 mark)*
Obtain consent *(1 mark)*

e *(1 mark for each correct answer, maximum 3 marks)*   /3
Previous tubal or pelvic surgery *(1 mark)*
PID *(1 mark)*
Endometriosis *(1 mark)*
IUCD in situ *(1 mark)*
Failed sterilisation *(1 mark)*
Previous ectopic pregnancy *(1 mark)*

Summary

The commonest site for an ectopic pregnancy to occur is within the fallopian tube, although pregnancies may also occur within the ovary or very rarely in the peritoneal cavity. Onset of symptoms may be sudden or gradual but any pain that is referred to the shoulder tip must be taken very seriously as it indicates tubal perforation. The only treatment for an ectopic pregnancy is surgical excision, possibly with removal of the fallopian tube if the contralateral tube is patent.

6 a *(1 mark for each correct answer, maximum 2 marks)*   /2
Cervical cancer *(1 mark)*
Cervical ectropion *(1 mark)*
Fibroids *(1 mark)*

b *(1 mark for each correct answer, maximum 3 marks)*   /3
Fertility – often reduced in endometriosis and
    fibroids *(1 mark)*
Dyspareunia – often accompanies endometriosis
    (1 mark)
Cycle length – often shorter with ovarian
    involvement of endometriosis *(1 mark)*
Menorrhagia can be a symptom of endometriosis
    and fibroids *(1 mark)*
Use of OCP – increases chances of ectropion
    (1 mark)
Family history of cervical cancer *(1 mark)*
Age of first sexual intercourse *(1 mark)*
Smear history *(1 mark)*

c *(1 mark for each correct answer, maximum 2 marks)*   /2
Fixed retroverted uterus *(1 mark)*
Adnexal mass *(1 mark)*
Thickening of uterosacral ligaments *(1 mark)*
Possible cystic swellings if ovaries involved *(1 mark)*

d *(1 mark for each correct answer, maximum 2 marks)*   /2
  FBC – anaemia *(1 mark)*
  TFTs – hypothyroidism is associated with
    menorrhagia *(1 mark)*
  Clotting – an abnormality can lead to increased
    blood loss *(1 mark)*
e *(maximum 1 mark)*   /1
  Perforation of bowel *(1 mark)*
  Perforation of major blood vessel *(1 mark)*

Summary

Endometriosis can affect any organ within the body and women may report pain that is disproportionate to the extent of their disease. Women with severe pain may have little disease on investigation and vice versa. Women with endometriosis may find conceiving a child more difficult and thus it might be worth referring them earlier for fertility investigations and assistance with conception.

7 a *(1 mark for each correct answer, maximum 2 marks)*   /2
  Depression *(1 mark)*
  Thyroid dysfunction *(1 mark)*
b *(1 mark for each correct answer, maximum 2 marks)*   /2
  TFTs *(1 mark)*
  FBC (to check Hb) *(1 mark)*
  LH : FSH ratio *(1 mark)*
c *(1 mark for each correct answer, maximum 2 marks)*   /2
  History of thromboembolism *(1 mark)*
  History of breast cancer *(1 mark)*
  History of migraines *(1 mark)*
d *(maximum 1 mark)*   /1
  A reduction in oestrogen levels causes vaginal
    atrophy and dryness *(1 mark)*. Lack of lubrication
    in the vagina causes discomfort during
    intercourse *(1 mark)*.
e *(1 mark for each correct answer, maximum 2 marks)*   /2
  Decreased libido *(1 mark)*
  Weight gain *(1 mark)*
  Loss of hair *(1 mark)*
  Mood swings *(1 mark)*
  Loss of energy *(1 mark)*

f *(1 mark for each correct answer, maximum 2 marks)*   `/2`
In a patient with an intact uterus, you must
prescribe a preparation which contains both
oestrogen and progesterone *(1 mark)*. The
progesterone is essential so that she has a
withdrawal bleed to shed the endometrium
each month *(1 mark)*. Otherwise her risk of
getting endometrial cancer is increased *(1 mark)*.
It must be explained that this will happen each
month.

Summary

The climacteric is the phase in a woman's life when she passes from
the reproductive to the non-reproductive phase. The menopause
is defined retrospectively as the last period a woman experiences.
Average age of menopause in Britain is 51. At the menopause
there will be high levels of LH, FSH and gonadotrophins as negative feedback is lost because the desensitised oocytes no longer
respond to stimulation by the gonadotrophins.

A woman is advised against taking HRT for more than 10 years
as after this time the risk of breast cancer is dramatically increases.
If the woman still wishes to continue it then this should be well
documented.

8 a Stress incontinence is the involuntary loss of urine   `/2`
during an increase in intra-abdominal pressure,
e.g. coughing, sneezing *(1 mark)*
Urge incontinence is a strong, sudden need to
urinate, followed by a bladder contraction,
which results in involuntary leakage *(1 mark)*

b *(1 mark for each correct answer, maximum 3 marks)*   `/3`
Previous pregnancy – especially if woman is a
multigravida or had large babies and difficult
vaginal deliveries *(1 mark)*
Prolapse *(1 mark)*
Menopause *(1 mark)*
Collagen disorders *(1 mark)*
Obesity *(1 mark)*

c *(maximum 1 mark)*   `/1`
Visible leakage of urine on coughing *(1 mark)*
Prolapse of the uterus *(1 mark)*

d *(1 mark for each correct answer, maximum 2 marks)* ☐ **/2**
    Pelvic floor exercises (patient has to be motivated to
       do these, have to be done a few times each day)
       (1 mark)
    Vaginal cones (the highest cone is placed in the
       vagina and woman learns to support it. When
       this is achieved a heavier cone is used) *(1 mark)*
    Topical oestrogens *(1 mark)*
    Ring or shelf pessary *(1 mark)*
e *(maximum 1 mark)* ☐ **/1**
    Burch colposuspension *(1 mark)*
    Insertion of a tension-free vaginal tape *(1 mark)*
f *(1 mark for each correct answer, maximum 2 marks)* ☐ **/2**
    Good surgical technique to support vaginal vault at
       hysterectomy *(1 mark)*
    Avoid prolonged second stage of labour *(1 mark)*
    Pelvic floor exercises after delivery *(1 mark)*
    HRT after menopause *(1 mark)*

Summary

There are three stages of uterine prolapse. First-degree prolapse is retroversion of the uterus and descent of the cervix within the vagina. If the cervix descends as far as the introitus it is described as second-degree. Third-degree prolapse is when the cervix and body of the uterus protrude through the introitus .This is also called 'procidentia'. In many of these women where there are co-morbidities present, surgical treatment is not an option but the condition is managed with pessaries and pelvic floor exercises.

9 a USS to determine exactly the gestation and ☐ **/1**
    location of the pregnancy *(1 mark)*
  b An anti-progesterone called mifepristone *(1 mark)* ☐ **/2**
    A prostaglandin called misoprostol *(1 mark)*
  c *(1 mark for each correct answer, maximum 3 marks)* ☐ **/3**
    Pregnancy of 64 days' gestation or over *(1 mark)*
    Suspected ectopic pregnancy *(1 mark)*
    Chronic hepatic/renal failure *(1 mark)*
    Severe asthma or COPD *(1 mark)*
    Long-term corticosteroid therapy *(1 mark)*
    Haemorrhagic disorders *(1 mark)*
    Patients with cardiovascular disease *(1 mark)*

d *(1 mark for each correct answer, maximum 3 marks)* `/3`
Haemorrhage *(1 mark)*
Uterine perforation *(1 mark)*
Cervical tears *(1 mark)*
Failure (continuing pregnancy) *(1 mark)*
Sepsis *(1 mark)*
Psychological trauma *(1 mark)*

e *(1 mark for each correct answer, maximum 3 marks)* `/3`
Early referral *(1 mark)*
Counselling *(1 mark)*
Offer a period of reflection *(1 mark)*
Patient information (verbal and written) *(1 mark)*
Screen for infection *(1 mark)*
Contraception counselling (might prevent a further termination in future) *(1 mark)*

Summary

A termination of pregnancy has to be done legally before 24 weeks' gestation. After this it can only be done if the life of the mother would be threatened if the pregnancy were to continue. After 24 weeks there is deemed to be a small but significant chance of independent survival from the mother, although the child often has various disabilities. Doctors should ensure advice is given about future contraception for these patients to prevent further unwanted pregnancy.

10 a *(1 mark for each correct answer, maximum 3 marks)* `/3`
Hypothyroidism *(1 mark)*
Endometriosis *(1 mark)*
Coagulopathy *(1 mark)*
Uterine polyps *(1 mark)*
Dysfunctional uterine bleeding *(1 mark)*

b *(1 mark for each correct answer, maximum 4 marks)* `/4`
Bleeding from other places *(1 mark)*
Bruising easily *(1 mark)*
Family history of coagulopathy *(1 mark)*
Any symptoms of hypothyroidism, e.g. recent weight gain, lethargy, constipation *(1 mark)*
Hirsutism *(1 mark)*
Acne *(1 mark)*
Is she diabetic *(1 mark)*

Dysmenorrhoea/pelvic pain *(1 mark)*
Dyspareunia *(1 mark)*

c *(1 mark for each correct answer, maximum 3 marks)* /3
LH : FSH ratio – increased *(1 mark)*
Serum androgen index – increased *(1 mark)*
Sex hormone binding globulin – decreased *(1 mark)*
Prolactin – increased *(1 mark)*
FBC – decreased Hb due to menorrhagia *(1 mark)*

d *(1 mark for each correct answer, maximum 2 marks)* /2
Infertility *(1 mark)*
Type 2 diabetes *(1 mark)*
Increased risk of endometrial hyperplasia and
    endometrial carcinoma *(1 mark)*
Increased risk of coronary heart disease *(1 mark)*

e *(1 mark for each correct answer, maximum 2 marks)* /2
Lose weight if obese *(1 mark)*
If normal weight, combined OCP for cycle control
    (1 mark)
Metformin can improve menstrual regularity by
    reducung insulin and free testosterone levels
    (1 mark)
Induction of ovulation with clomiphene *(1 mark)*

Summary

Patients may present with a range of symptoms, from menorrhagia and hirsutism, to infertility. The diagnosis of polycystic ovarian syndrome is based on a transvaginal US scan and hormone profile including measurement of FSH/LH and testosterone. PCOS accounts for 80% of cases of oligomenorrhoea. Metformin can be used to help with weight loss, and induce regular periods, with contraceptive advice needed as ovulation may restart. The cosmetic symptoms can be more devastating for the patient than the physical symptoms and these should be dealt with sensitively.

17 Orthopaedics

QUESTIONS

1 Oscar, an 18-year-old boy felt his knee 'pop' whilst playing football last week. He has had pain in his knee since then, and it appears to catch from time to time. Yesterday his knee locked, and he couldn't straighten or bend it without having to massage his joint.

    a What is the most likely diagnosis?   *1 mark*
    b Name one specific test for this condition.   *1 mark*
    c List three of the functions of the meniscus.   *3 marks*
    d What investigation would you request for this patient?   *1 mark*
    e What basic treatment and advice would you give this patient?   *4 marks*
    f Name one surgical treatment of this condition.   *1 mark*

2 Erica, a 17-year-old girl, injured her anterior cruciate ligament whilst skiing.

    a Give two early and one late symptom of an ACL tear.   *3 marks*
    b What causes an ACL tear?   *1 mark*
    c Name two examinations that may show an abnormality in this patient.   *2 marks*
    d What single investigation would you request to confirm the diagnosis?   *1 mark*
    e What surgical option is there for this patient?   *1 mark*
    f Give three possible complications of an arthroscopy.   *3 marks*

3 Miss Brundwell, a 32-year-old GP, was hit on the side of the leg by a car whilst out jogging.

    a Is this a varus or valgus injury?   *1 mark*
    b What is the most likely ligament injured in the course of this accident?   *1 mark*

Complete SAQs for Medical Finals By P. Stather et al, Published 2010 by
Blackwell Publishing, ISBN: 978-1-4501-8928-6.

    c Give three symptoms of this condition.   *3 marks*

    d Explain how you would perform a thorough
       examination of the knee.   *5 marks*

4 Tania, a 7-year-old girl, was playing on top of a climbing frame
  when she tripped and fell off the frame onto her left arm.

    a Which two types of fractures occur only in
       children?   *2 marks*

    b List the three typical signs and symptoms of
       a fracture.   *3 marks*

    c Give four aspects of your management of this
       patient.   *4 marks*

    d Suggest two pieces of advice you would give to
       this patient and her parents to help prevent
       further accidents.   *2 marks*

    e Give three features which might make you
       suspect non-accidental injury.   *3 marks*

5 Dr Foster, a 45-year-old surgeon, had been noticing pain in his
  right shoulder for the past 3 weeks. It is most prominent when
  he attempts to serve whilst playing tennis, and reaching for
  objects on a high shelf.

    a Name the muscles of the rotator cuff.   *4 marks*

    b What might you see on inspection of this
       patient's shoulder?   *2 marks*

    c Give two other symptoms you may elicit during
       the examination.   *2 marks*

    d Name one special examination which would be
       positive in this case.   *1 mark*

    e Which two other joints would you examine in
       this patient?   *2 marks*

6 Hope, a 30-year-old secretary, has been diagnosed with supraspinatus tendonitis.

    a What is the common name for this condition?   *1 mark*

    b State the range of movement during which
       there is likely to be pain in this patient.   *2 marks*

    c What is the cause of the pain in this condition?   *2 marks*

    d What is the innervation of supraspinatus?   *2 marks*

    e Explain three ways that this condition may be
       managed.   *3 marks*

7 A 73-year-old lady comes into A & E after falling on some ice outside her house. She slipped and put her arm out to protect herself. Apart from feeling a bit bruised she complains of pain in her right wrist. You order an x-ray as you suspect a Colles fracture.

   a Give three features you might see on x-ray.   ***3 marks***

   b What is the name given to the fracture caused by falling with the wrist flexed?   ***1 mark***

   c Outline your examination of the wrist.   ***4 marks***

   d The x-ray comes back and you diagnose a Colles fracture. Along with a Colles fracture, suggest two other accompanying fractures you would be looking for.   ***2 marks***

   e The fracture is not displaced. How would you treat this?   ***2 marks***

   f Name two long-term complications of a Colles fracture apart from associated fractures.   ***2 marks***

8 A 14-year-old obese boy comes to see his GP with pain in his right hip that spreads to his groin and knee. It is worse when he runs but is there on walking. It has become so bad that he has had to be excused from PE at school. Previously his GP said that it was growing pains but his mother is worried and has brought him to you for a second opinion. You suspect SUFE.

   a Apart from SUFE, what are the two most likely differential diagnoses?   ***2 marks***

   b What three features in the history are consistent with SUFE?   ***3 marks***

   c What two features would you look for to confirm your thinking?   ***2 marks***

   d Briefly outline the pathophysiology of the condition.   ***2 marks***

   e Give two ways you would manage the patient in the GP surgery.   ***2 marks***

   f Suggest two complications of this condition.   ***2 marks***

9 An 86-year-old lady comes to A & E after being found lying on the floor by a neighbour. She did not bang her head or lose consciousness. Her left hip is very painful and she required assistance to get up. You suspect there may be a fracture.

   a Give two features, consistent with your suspicions, that you would look for on examination.   ***2 marks***

  b Apart from examining the hip, what else would
     you do in terms of examination?   *2 marks*
  c Give three investigations you would request for
     this patient.   *3 marks*
  d What is the blood supply to the femoral head?   *3 marks*
  e Give two consequences of avascular necrosis.   *2 marks*
  f The orthopaedic surgeon performs an operation to
     fix the hip fracture. The following day the
     physiotherapist mobilises the patient. Why is this
     so important?   *3 marks*

10 A 52-year-old man comes to your orthopaedic outpatient clinic. He has a long history of osteoarthritis in both knees. He says that the pain is getting worse despite complying with conservative treatments. He is reluctant to leave the house because the pain is so bad.

  a Give three conservative measures he might
     have been told to try.   *3 marks*
     The patient is keen to have a bilateral joint
     replacement as a friend of his had this done and
     has been impressed by the results. However, you
     feel that your patient is rather young to have this
     operation and would like to try other measures
     first to help his pain, as so far only over-the-
     counter preparations have been used.
  b What else can you do for the pain?   *2 marks*
  c He goes away having tried these and returns
     9 months later saying that these are no longer
     helping. Apart from a joint replacement, what
     two other surgical procedures could be
     performed for this patient?   *2 marks*
  d In what three other conditions might be a joint
     replacement eventually be appropriate?   *3 marks*
  e Suggest four complications that can develop after
     a joint replacement.   *4 marks*

11 A boy of 5 comes to your outpatient clinic with his mother. He has been walking with a limp off and on for 4 months now and complains of pain in his left hip. The GP asked for a hip x-ray but no untoward changes were seen. You suspect Perthe's disease.

  a Outline the pathophysiology of Perthe's disease.   *2 marks*
  b Give two differential diagnoses.   *2 marks*

c What investigation would you do to confirm
your diagnosis, given that a recent x-ray was
normal? *1 mark*

d Give two radiological changes you would expect
in established disease. *2 marks*

e Your suspicions are confirmed and your
investigations suggest Perthe's disease. You treat
your patient conservatively without surgery and
continue to monitor him regularly. Name three
adverse prognostic indicators. *3 marks*

Orthopaedics

ANSWERS

1 a Meniscal tear *(1 mark)* `/1`
  b *(maximum 1 mark)* `/1`
    McMurray's test *(1 mark)*
    Apley's test *(1 mark)*
  c *(1 mark for each correct answer, maximum 3 marks)* `/3`
    Buffer between the joint *(1 mark)*
    Shock absorption system *(1 mark)*
    Lubrication *(1 mark)*
    Limits flexion and extension *(1 mark)*
  d *(maximum 1 mark)* `/1`
    MRI knee *(1 mark)*
    Arthroscopy *(1 mark)*
  e *(1 mark for each correct answer, maximum 4 marks)* `/4`
    Knee immobiliser *(1 mark)*
    Ice *(1 mark)*
    NSAIDs *(1 mark)*
    Do not fully weight bear *(1 mark)*
    Advice about sports *(1 mark)*
    Advice to return if no improvement *(1 mark)*
  f *(maximum 1 mark)* `/1`
    Meniscal repair *(1 mark)*
    Meniscectomy *(1 mark)*

Summary

Meniscal tears are common sporting injuries, classically appearing as bucket handle tears. They tend to cause pain and locking of the joint, with giving way and minimal swelling. If rapid massive swelling does occur this is indicative of a haemarthrosis, which should be rapidly investigated and treated.

2 a *(1 mark for each correct answer, maximum 3 marks)* `/3`
    Early – pain *(1 mark)*, swelling *(1 mark)*
    Late – arthritis *(1 mark)*, joint instability *(1 mark)*

b Hyperextension and inversion of the knee *(1 mark)* `/1`

c *(1 mark for each correct answer, maximum 2 marks)* `/2`
  Anterior drawer test *(1 mark)*
  Lachman's test *(1 mark)*
  Pivot shift test *(1 mark)*

d MRI knee *(1 mark)* `/1`

e ACL reconstruction using a graft *(1 mark)*, `/1`
  typically from the patellar tendon. A repair is
  not possible.

f *(1 mark for each correct answer, maximum 3 marks)* `/3`
  DVT *(1 mark)*
  Infection *(1 mark)*
  Excessive bleeding *(1 mark)*
  Anaesthetic reaction *(1 mark)*
  Damage to cartilage *(1 mark)*
  Paraesthesia over knee *(1 mark)*

Summary

Anterior cruciate ligament injury is the most common form of ligamentous injury. It is due to external rotation of the tibia on the femur, which occurs most commonly in sporting events. Treatment is usually conservative with extensive physiotherapy to strengthen the hamstrings; however, surgery can be used, particularly if the patient wishes to continue their sporting activities.

3 a Valgus *(1 mark)* `/1`

b Medial collateral ligament *(1 mark)* `/1`

c *(1 mark for each correct answer, maximum 3 marks)* `/3`
  Pain *(1 mark)*
  Swelling *(1 mark)*
  Joint stiffness *(1 mark)*
  Joint instability *(1 mark)*

d *(1 mark for each correct answer, maximum 5 marks)* `/5`
  Look for scars, deformity, swelling *(1 mark)*
  Palpate for any tenderness or effusion *(1 mark)*
  Assess movement of the joint *(1 mark)*
  Perform the special tests such as anterior and
    posterior drawer, Lachman's, pivot shift, varus
    and valgus stress, McMurray's test, and Apley's
    test *(1 mark per special test named, maximum
    2 marks)*

Summary
The medial collateral ligament is more commonly injured than the lateral as it is less mobile, and is often associated with fractures of the tibial plateau. In severe cases the common peroneal nerve may also be damaged, resulting in foot drop.

4 a Greenstick fracture *(1 mark)*   `/2`
Salter-Harris epiphyseal fractures *(1 mark)*

  b Pain *(1 mark)*   `/3`
Swelling *(1 mark)*
Deformity *(1 mark)*

  c *(1 mark for each correct answer, maximum 4 marks)*   `/4`
X-ray *(1 mark)*
Rest *(1 mark)*
Ice *(1 mark)*
Compress *(1 mark)*
Elevate *(1 mark)*
Plaster cast *(1 mark)*

  d *(1 mark for each correct answer, maximum*   `/2`
2 marks)
Encourage regular exercise and a healthy diet to
build strong healthy bones *(1 mark)*
Wear safety equipment *(1 mark)*
Appropriate supervision *(1 mark)*

  e *(1 mark for each correct answer, maximum 3 marks)*   `/3`
Fractures in immobile children *(1 mark)*
Inconsistent story *(1 mark)*
Delayed presentation *(1 mark)*
Repeated injuries *(1 mark)*
Recurrent admissions *(1 mark)*
Injury out of context of age of patient *(1 mark)*
Withdrawn child *(1 mark)*
Child appears scared of guardian *(1 mark)*

Summary
Greenstick fractures are confined to the more malleable bones. The bone ends remain in opposition, but angulation is possible. They tend to heal well and rapidly.

5 a Supraspinatus *(1 mark)*   `/4`
Infraspinatus *(1 mark)*

Subscapularis *(1 mark)*
Teres minor *(1 mark)*
b Muscular atrophy of the deltoid causing
    asymmetry *(1 mark)*   /2
Swelling *(1 mark)*
c Pain and weakness on extension and abduction,   /2
    and internal and external rotation of
    the arm *(1 mark)*
Crepitus over the shoulder joint *(1 mark)*
d *(maximum 1 mark)*   /1
Hawkin's test *(1 mark)*
Drop arm test for impingement *(1 mark)*
e Neck *(1 mark)*   /2
Elbow *(1 mark)*

Summary

Rotator cuff injuries are often due to repetitive stress, and tend to heal with rest, ice and support. Supraspinatus is the most commonly injured muscle, causing localised pain under the anterior aspect of the clavicle. For persistent cases intra-articular injections of steroids may be used, prior to surgical investigation of the joint.

6 a Painful arc syndrome *(1 mark)*   /1
  b 70–120 degrees during active abduction *(1 mark)*   /2
  c The supraspinatus tendon impinges *(1 mark)*   /2
    under the acromion *(1 mark)*
  d Suprascapular nerve *(1 mark)*, C5/6 *(1 mark)*   /2
  e *(1 mark for each correct answer, maximum 3 marks)* /3
    Conservatively with rest, ice and physiotherapy to
      allow the inflammation to settle *(1 mark)*
    Medically with NSAIDs, or a corticosteroid injection
      into the joint *(1 mark for either example)*
    Surgically with an arthroscopic acromioplasty, or
      repair of the rotator cuff tendons *(1 mark for either
      example)*

Summary

Supraspinatus tendonitis is a common cause of shoulder restriction at all ages. It commonly follows trauma, and causes pain in the shoulder radiating to the upper arm. On examination the joint may be immobilised due to pain, however passive movements are easier, and there may be spasm of the trapezius muscle.

7 a *(1 mark for each correct answer, maximum 3 marks)* `/3`
  Dorsal displacement of the distal fragment *(1 mark)*
  The shaft of the radius is driven into the distal
    fragment leading to impaction *(1 mark)*
  Ulnar angulation *(1 mark)*
  The fracture can be displaced giving a 'dinner fork'
    deformity *(1 mark)*
b Smith's fracture *(1 mark)* `/1`
c *(1 mark for each correct answer, maximum 4 marks)* `/4`
  Inspection – swelling, deformity *(1 mark)*
  Palpation – of bone and joints, can any tenderness
    be elicited? *(1 mark)*
  Nerves – sensation *(1 mark)*
  Blood vessels – pulses, warmth *(1 mark)*
  Movement may be painful *(1 mark)*
d *(1 mark for each correct answer, maximum 2 marks)* `/3`
  Ulnar styloid *(1 mark)*
  Radial head *(1 mark)*
  Scaphoid *(1 mark)*
e Apply a plaster cast with the hand (distal fragment) `/2`
    in palmer flexion and ulnar deviation *(1 mark)*
  Keep on for 6 weeks and then fracture clinic
    appointment *(1 mark)*
f *(1 mark for each correct answer, maximum 2 marks)* `/2`
  Carpal tunnel syndrome *(1 mark)*
  Persisting stiffness *(1 mark)*
  Delayed rupture of extensor pollicis longus *(1 mark)*.
    The tendon is weakened by the roughness at the
    fracture site.
  Malunion causing pain in the distal radio-ulnar joint
    and decreased supination *(1 mark)*
  Prominence of the distal ulna *(1 mark)*

Summary
If displacement is present, the reduction is checked with x-rays, with the neurovascular supply and fixation reviewed the following day. While the limb is in plaster the shoulder and fingers must be exercised to maintain mobility and muscle strength. The cast must stay on for 6 weeks until the fracture has united.

8 a *(1 mark for each correct answer, maximum 2 marks)* `/2`
   Perthe's disease *(1 mark)*
   Osteomyelitis *(1 mark)*
   Traumatic hip fracture *(1 mark)*

b Male *(1 mark)* `/3`
   14 years old *(1 mark)*
   Obese *(1 mark)*

c *(1 mark for each correct answer, maximum 2 marks)* `/2`
   Right leg externally rotated and 1–2 cm shorter
      than the left *(1 mark)*
   Decreased range of abduction and internal rotation
      (1 mark)
   After an acute slip all hip movements are painful
      (1 mark)

d *(1 mark for each correct answer, maximum 2 marks)* `/2`
   During the pre-pubertal growth spurt, the
   relatively immature physis of the proximal femur
   is too weak to resist the increased stress on it by
   the increase in body weight *(1 mark)*. There is an
   imbalance between pituitary hormones
   stimulating bone growth and gonadal hormone,
   which encourages physeal fusion *(1 mark)*. Hence
   it is usually seen in obese or tall and thin
   adolescents *(1 mark)*. It can also be caused by
   trauma *(1 mark)*

e *(1 mark for each correct answer, maximum 2 marks)* `/2`
   Lateral and AP x-rays of hip and knee *(1 mark)*
   Orthopaedic referral *(1 mark)*
   Analgesia *(1 mark)*
   Advise abstinence from exercise until orthopaedics
      review *(1 mark)*

f *(1 mark for each correct answer, maximum 2 marks)* `/2`
   Coxa vara deformity *(1 mark)*
   Slipping of the opposite hip happens in 1/3 cases
      (1 mark)
   Secondary osteoarthritis *(1 mark)*
   Chronic pain *(1 mark)*

Summary

Slipped upper femoral epiphysis tends to occur in overweight boys
in their early teenage years. It causes the patient to limp due to

a painful joint, an externally rotated and shortened leg, with a decreased range of movements.

9 a *(1 mark for each correct answer, maximum 2 marks)* /2

If she can bear weight through it *(1 mark)*

Lateral rotation of left leg *(1 mark)*

Shortening of left leg *(1 mark)*

All hip movements to be painful *(1 mark)*

b *(1 mark for each correct answer, maximum 2 marks)* /2

Primary survey looking for other injuries *(1 mark)*

Full neurological examination – did she have a TIA/ stroke that made her fall *(1 mark)*

Auscultate heart – is there a murmur that gave rise to an arrhythmia that caused a syncope. *(1 mark)*

c Bloods – FBC, U+E, CRP, calcium levels, clotting, group and save (in case an operation is needed), glucose *(maximum 1 mark)* /3

Dip urine for infection *(1 mark)*

AP and lateral X-ray views of left hip and knee (there may be an associated fracture further down the femoral shaft) *(1 mark)*

d Vessels in the ligament of the head of femur (ligamentum teres) *(1 mark)* /3

Medial circumflex femoral arteries *(1 mark)*

Nutrient vessels in the substance of the bone *(1 mark)*

e *(1 mark for each correct answer, maximum 2 marks)* /2

The fracture may fail to unite *(1 mark)*

Collapse of the articular space leads to osteoarthritis *(1 mark)*

Chronic pain *(1 mark)*

Hip joint replacement *(1 mark)*

f *(1 mark for each correct answer, maximum 3 marks)* /3

Being bed-bound increases the risk of DVT *(1 mark)*, pneumonia *(1 mark)* and pressure sores *(1 mark)*. Early mobilisation prevents these from occurring.

The earlier she mobilises the sooner she can go home, freeing up an acute care bed and reducing the cost of her hospital stay *(1 mark)*

Increases blood supply to the joint to aid faster heeling *(1 mark)*

Summary

Osteoporosis is the most important predisposing factor for fractures, which is usually seen in postmenopausal women. Its severity increases with age. In the younger population osteoporosis is sometimes secondary to chronic alcoholism, or steroid use.

X-rays for fractured NOF should always include the pelvis as pain in the hip and difficulty weight bearing may be due to a fracture of the pubic ramus rather than a fractured NOF.

10 a *(1 mark for each correct answer, maximum 3 marks)* `/3`
Lose weight *(1 mark)*
Walking stick/aid *(1 mark)*
NSAIDs *(1 mark)*
Exercise to keep the joints supple *(1 mark)*
Physiotherapy/OT *(1 mark)*

b *(1 mark for each correct answer, maximum 2 marks)* `/2`
Injections of hyaluronic acid derivatives *(1 mark)*
  – they provide cushioning to the knee
Intra-articular injections of hydrocortisone
  (1 mark) – reduce inflammation
Stronger prescription painkillers such as codeine
  (1 mark)

c *(1 mark for each correct answer, maximum 2 marks)* `/2`
Debridement of the joint *(1 mark)* – done
  arthroscopically to remove loose pieces of
  cartilage and debris that can cause irritation
Osteotomy *(1 mark)* – realigning bones
Arthrodesis *(1 mark)* – fusing bones, a less viable
  option because the joint has no flexibility

d *(1 mark for each correct answer, maximum 3 marks)* `/3`
Rheumatoid arthritis *(1 mark)*
Osteoporosis *(1 mark)*
Avascular necrosis of the femoral head *(1 mark)*
Metastatic lesions and pathological fractures *(1 mark)*
Trauma *(1 mark)*

e *(1 mark for each correct answer, maximum 4 marks)* `/4`
Infection – osteomyelitis *(1 mark)*
DVT *(1 mark)*
Pressure sores *(1 mark)*
Loosening of implant *(1 mark)*
Fat embolism *(1 mark)* – part of the marrow can
  get into the circulation

Problems with wound healing *(1 mark)*

Bleeding *(1 mark)* – can lead to haematoma
formation

Numbness around part of the wound *(1 mark)*

Nerve damage *(1 mark)* – e.g. foot drop after a knee
replacement

Decreased range of movement *(1 mark)*

Summary

Joint replacements are increasingly common. Their lifespan is about 15 years but this can vary depending on the stresses the joint is put under. They are reserved for older people as they would need to be replaced more frequently in younger people. Alternatives to joint replacement include joint resurfacing which can postpone the need for a replacement.

11 a *(1 mark for each correct answer, maximum 2 marks)* **/2**

It is caused by temporary loss of blood supply
to the hip. The head of the femur starts to die,
becoming ischaemic. *(1 mark)*

The blood supply to the femoral head changes
during childhood *(1 mark)*. At around age
4 the metaphyseal supply has ceased and
by age 7 the vessels in the ligamentum teres
have developed *(1 mark)*. Between these
ages the blood supply can be compromised
(1 mark)

b *(1 mark for each correct answer, maximum 2 marks)* **/2**

Irritable hip *(1 mark)*

Attention seeking *(1 mark)*

Soft tissue injury *(1 mark)*

c Bone scan *(1 mark)* **/1**

X-rays can appear normal at first in the course
of the disease *(1 mark)*

d Flattened femoral head when its appearance **/2**
should be rounded *(1 mark)*

A broken or damaged femoral head *(1 mark)*

e Older age of onset *(1 mark)* – if the child is **/3**
younger there is more scope for the bone to
grow and remodel naturally before the child
stops growing.

Gender *(1 mark)* – girls generally do worse than boys as boys finish growing at a later age than girls do.

Severity *(1 mark)* – the more severe the condition (x-ray changes are a good indicator), the worse the prognosis as there is a greater risk of persisting difficulties.

Summary

Severity of Perthe's disease is classified on the Catterall grading of Perthe's disease scale. Grade 1 is the lowest grade with cyst formation in the anterolateral aspect of the epiphysis. Grade 4 is where the whole of the head is involved. This grade has the poorest prognosis.

18 General Surgery

QUESTIONS

1 A 23-year-old girl is admitted to SAU with right iliac fossa pain and vomiting.

   a What four further questions would you like to ask to try to establish a diagnosis?   ***4 marks***

   b Name three differential diagnoses apart from appendicitis.   ***3 marks***

   c You suspect appendicitis. Suggest two abnormalities you will be expecting to find on examination.   ***2 marks***

   d You are the house officer on call. Give three aspects of your initial management.   ***3 marks***

   e Occasionally appendicitis can present after it has become walled off by omentum. What is this called?   ***1 mark***

2 A 55-year-old lady is admitted to SAU with right upper quadrant pain. It has been there as a dull ache for a week but is much more severe today. The pain was made worse by eating fish and chips for dinner. You diagnose cholecystitis.

   a Name three risk factors for developing cholecystitis.   ***3 marks***

   b What are the main two components of gallstones?   ***2 marks***

   c What is the name given to the pain that is caused by a gallstone obstructing the neck of the gallbladder?   ***1 mark***

   d What percentage of gallstones are radiolucent?   ***1 mark***

   e What two investigations would you order for this patient?   ***2 marks***

   f Apart from pain, name three complications of gallstones.   ***3 marks***

Complete SAQs for Medical Finals By P. Stather et al, Published 2010 by Blackwell Publishing. ISBN: 978-1-4501-8928-6.

3 A 65-year-old lady arrived at A & E with right upper quadrant and epigastric pain. Her pain is worse on movement. She has a temperature of 38.7°C, and has vomited a few times today. She has a history of gallstones and has been treated conservatively for this in the past.

    a You examine her and elicit Murphy's sign. Describe this and explain the result.   *2 marks*

    b What two investigations would you order and what you expect them to show?   *2 marks*

    c What is the treatment of acute cholecystitis?   *2 marks*

    d Although this will treat the initial episode, what is the ultimate treatment for gallstones/cholecystitis?   *1 mark*

    e Give two advantages of a laparoscopic procedure.   *2 marks*

    f A scan shows that there is a small gallstone in the common bile duct and blood tests show a picture of obstructive jaundice. How can the stone be removed from the bile duct?   *1 mark*

    g Why is it important to remove the stone?   *2 marks*

4 A 40-year-old woman comes to see you due to unsightly bulging veins in both of her legs. They cause her pain at work as she is standing most of the day as a hairdresser.

    a What is the definition of varicose veins?   *1 mark*

    b Name three risk factors for developing this condition.   *3 marks*

    c Briefly outline their aetiology.   *2 marks*

    d Name two popular sites where valves can become incompetent.   *2 marks*

    e Name three features which may be found on the legs of a patient who has varicose veins.   *3 marks*

    f Your patient is very distressed at the cosmetic appearance of her varicose veins. What treatments could you offer her?   *2 marks*

    g Before offering a female patient of this age a surgical procedure what would you want to discuss with her first?   *1 mark*

5 A 60-year-old man comes to see you having been experiencing pain in his lower left leg when walking to the shops. He can walk about 100 yards before the pain comes on and is relieved by rest for a few minutes. He describes the pain as a cramp.

a   What is the name given to this condition?   *1 mark*
b   Give three risk factors for his condition.   *3 marks*
c   How would you treat this patient to improve
    his condition?   *2 marks*
d   After 2 years this patient comes to see you
    again. His pain has not improved and he now
    gets pain in bed at night in his left foot.
    He can only walk 30 yards before having stop
    due to pain. You notice his left foot appears
    red in colour compared to his right.
    Co-codamol tablets prescribed by his GP are
    not helping with the pain. Why do patients
    get pain at night when blood supply to the limb
    is minimal?   *2 marks*
e   What three investigations would you order?   *3 marks*
f   The symptoms are affecting the patient's life and
    he describes life as being 'unbearable'. Your
    investigations show he has a 70% narrowing of
    his lower femoral artery. Suggest three possible
    treatment options.   *3 marks*

6   A 26-year-old man comes to SAU with pain around his lower
    back region that has been tender for about 10 days. He went to
    see his GP who prescribed antibiotics 3 days ago for an abscess
    but they have not helped. He is in a lot of pain now. You exam-
    ine him and diagnose a pilonidal abscess.
    a   What is the most common anatomical location
        for this?   *1 mark*
    b   Briefly outline the aetiology of a pilonidal sinus.   *1 mark*
    c   Name two common organisms which infect
        the sinus.   *2 marks*
    d   Give two factors thought to be associated with
        an increased risk of developing pilonidal sinus.   *2 marks*
    e   What is the surgical management in i) an
        emergency, ii) electively?   *2 marks*
    f   What is the recurrence rate for this condition?   *1 mark*
    g   Name the two different types of wound healing.   *2 marks*

7   A 70-year-old male presents to you with a lump in his right
    groin. He first noticed it 6 months ago when he was standing
    brushing his teeth in the morning. It was not noticeable when
    he woke up and was lying in bed. He said that he is able to push

the lump back in himself but this has become more difficult recently. It is not painful. You diagnose an indirect inguinal hernia.

a What is the difference between a direct and
   an indirect inguinal hernia?   *2 marks*
b Name two risk factors for the development
   of a hernia.   *2 marks*
c Name the borders of the inguinal canal.   *4 marks*
d You offer your patient a laparoscopic hernia
   repair. Name two complications of this procedure. *2 marks*
e When a patient presents with a lump in the
   groin what three other differential diagnoses
   should you consider?   *3 marks*
f Describe what is meant by a 'strangulated' hernia. *1 mark*

8 An 83-year-old lady presents to SAU with severe abdominal pain and vomiting. She has very little past medical history and is normally fit and well. She had an appendicectomy as a child.

a What four questions would you like to ask?   *4 marks*
b You request an abdominal x-ray and find
   that she has a large bowel obstruction.
   Why would you also have requested an erect
   chest x-ray?   *1 mark*
c Name three possible causes of a bowel obstruction. *3 marks*
d Conservative measures to resolve her obstruction
   do not help and you decide to take her down to
   theatre for laparotomy. On the table you discover
   she has a large tumour of her descending colon.
   What is the staging system for colorectal cancer
   and briefly outline each stage.   *4 marks*
e Name two risk factors for colorectal cancer.   *2 marks*

9 A 34-year-old man presents with a lump in his right testicle that is not painful. He noticed it by accident in the shower one morning. You suspect it might be a tumour.

a What are the two types of germ cell tumour?   *1 mark*
b What two features on examination would you
   be looking for that would suggest it is a testicular
   tumour?   *2 marks*
c Apart from examining the lump, what two other
   areas would you examine on this patient?   *2 marks*
d What two blood tests would you request?   *2 marks*

    e You investigate the patient with an USS and
biopsy which show this is malignant and an
orchidectomy is performed. A whole-body
CT scan shows that the cancer has not spread.
Suggest four areas of your management of this
patient now. *4 marks*

10 A 13-year-old boy presents to A & E with pain in his scrotum
and groin on the left side. It started 2 hours ago and has not
relented despite taking ibuprofen.

    a Apart from torsion of the left testicle name two
other differential diagnoses. *2 marks*

    b Suggest three ways in which you could
distinguish between these diagnoses. *3 marks*

    c You decide to take him to theatre urgently to explore
the possibility of a torsion. Why is it important to
act sooner rather than later in this case? *1 mark*

    d Before taking the patient to theatre, state one
complication you must warn the patient about
specific to this operation, which you should obtain
his consent for? *1 mark*

    e What is a risk factor for torsion? *1 mark*

    f Give three other symptoms/signs you would
need to be present for you to make a diagnosis
of epidymo-orchitis. *3 marks*

    g Give two risk factors for epididymo-orchitis. *2 marks*

11 A 37-year-old woman notices a small but firm lump on her
right breast one morning in the shower. It is not painful. She
has no previous history of breast problems.

    a What three diagnoses would you consider? *3 marks*

    b What four further questions might you ask her? *4 marks*

    c On examination you find a hard 2 cm lump in
the inner lower quadrant of her left breast. It is
smooth to the touch and rubbery in texture.
It moves easily under the skin. What is the
likely diagnosis now? *1 mark*

    d Give two ways you would investigate
this patient. *2 marks*

    e What follow-up care will this patient need,
if your suspected diagnosis is correct? *1 mark*

    f Is her risk of breast cancer increased? *1 mark*

12 A 55-year-old lady presents to her GP with a painless lump in her breast. She noticed it 4 weeks ago but had been too busy at work to come and see you. Now she has noticed her nipple appears to have become drawn in. This morning she noticed a drop of blood in her bra.

    a What four further points would you elicit in the history?   *4 marks*

    b Tru-cut biopsy shows cancerous cells. What are the next two steps in this patient's work-up?   *2 marks*

    c What is the difference between stage and grade of a tumour?   *2 marks*

    d What three other treatments might this patient be eligible for?   *3 marks*

    e Give two areas breast cancer commonly metastasises to.   *2 marks*

13 A 17-year-old girl is admitted to SAU with right loin pain radiating into her back. She was diagnosed with UTI by her GP 3 days ago and was prescribed cefalexin. This has not helped and her pain has worsened. She has a prior medical history of diabetes mellitus.

    a Suggest your four initial investigations.   *4 marks*

    b You diagnose pyelonephritis. Her observations are: temp. 38.7°C, HR 110, BP 92/60. She is vomiting and feeling very unwell. Give four steps in your management of this acute condition.   *4 marks*

    c Suggest two ways you would manage this patient in the long term.   *2 marks*

    d Name two factors that predispose a person to develop pyelonephritis.   *2 marks*

14 A 67-year-old woman comes into SAU with severe epigastric pain that radiates to the back. She finds that sitting forwards helps ease the pain rather than lying flat. She is vomiting. You suspect pancreatitis.

    a What three initial investigations would you perform and why?   *3 marks*

    b Name four causes of pancreatitis.   *4 marks*

    c Outline three aspects of your management as an FY1 doctor.   *3 marks*

    d Name two early and two late complications of pancreatitis.   *4 marks*

15 Frank is 58. He is a retired headteacher who was forced to retire due to ill health. He has suffered from diabetes for 11 years and in the last three years he has been admitted increasingly frequently. Today he is admitted after having been found collapsed on the floor at his home. He is conscious and denies any chest pain. Observations are: HR 134, BP 94/48, resp. 28, temp. 38.6°C. There is no obvious source for his sepsis until, on removing his socks, you find a large ulcer on his heel.

   a Name three types of ulcers.   *3 marks*

   b Give two features used to identify each of the above ulcers.   *3 marks*

   c After examining Frank you discover he has reduced sensation in both feet extending to the midcalves on both legs. Suggest two ways of investigating him further.   *2 marks*

   d Once he is feeling better Frank mentions that he spends all day sitting as he cannot walk far due to pain in his legs which extends to his buttocks. What is this called, and what is the name of the syndrome which includes leg pain, buttock pain and impotence?   *2 marks*

   e Explain the pathology behind the development of varicose veins.   *2 marks*

16 Bruce, a 57-year-old male, presents with a 7-day history of severe left iliac fossa pain, fever and vomiting and reports that he has not opened his bowels for 3 days. On examination he is tachycardic with tenderness, rebound and guarding in the left iliac fossa.

   a You suspect diverticular disease. Explain what diverticular disease is.   *2 marks*

   b Name two risk factors for diverticular disease.   *2 marks*

   c Give two steps in the management of acute diverticulitis.   *2 marks*

   d He tells you that he is allergic to penicillin. Name two alternatives you can prescribe.   *1 mark*

   e Constipation is a very common problem. Give five other causes of constipation.   *5 marks*

17 Arthur, a 62-year-old male, presents to you with several months' history of weight loss and rectal bleeding. You suspect a malignancy.

a What further symptoms would you
  enquire about? Name four. *4 marks*
b Name two risk factors for colorectal cancer. *2 marks*
c Name two investigations apart from a blood
  test you would request. *2 marks*
d Arthur successfully undergoes surgery to
  remove his tumour and a stoma is sited.
  Give three complications of a stoma *3 marks*

18 Caroline, a 25-year-old lady, who is currently 34 weeks pregnant with her first child, presents to her GP with rectal bleeding. She has passed moderate quantities of bright red blood that covers her stools. She has pain when passing stools.

a Name the most likely condition. *1 mark*
b Other than pregnancy, give two risk factors
  for this condition. *2 marks*
c What two symptoms may she have? *2 marks*
d How is the severity of this condition classified?
  Give a brief description of each. *3 marks*
e Give four ways that this condition can
  be treated. *4 marks*

General Surgery

ANSWERS

1 a *(1 mark for each correct answer, maximum 4 marks)* `/4`
  Has pain always been in RIF or did it start more
    centrally? *(1 mark)*
  What stage of menstrual cycle is she in? *(1 mark)*
  Any lower urinary tract symptoms? *(1 mark)*
  Any change in bowel habit? *(1 mark)*
  Was the pain acute in onset or gradual? *(1 mark)*
  Fever? *(1 mark)*
  Any PV bleeding? *(1 mark)*

b *(1 mark for each correct answer, maximum 3 marks)* `/3`
  Right-sided ectopic pregnancy *(1 mark)*
  Torsion of a right-sided ovarian cyst *(1 mark)*
  UTI *(1 mark)*
  Gastroenteritis *(1 mark)*

c Rebound tenderness *(1 mark)* `/2`
  Guarding *(1 mark)*

d *(1 mark for each correct answer, maximum 3 marks)* `/3`
  Admit *(1 mark)*
  NBM *(1 mark)*
  IV fluids *(1 mark)*
  Bloods – FBC, CRP, U+E *(maximum 1 mark)*
  Urine dip *(1 mark)*
  Pregnancy test *(1 mark)*
  Senior review *(1 mark)*
  Analgesia *(1 mark)*
  Anti-emetic *(1 mark)*

e Appendix mass *(1 mark)* `/1`

Summary

An inflamed appendix is always a differential diagnosis of RIF pain. Diagnosis is clinical, based on clinical signs of guarding and rebound tenderness, pyrexia and a raised WCC and CRP. The only confirmation is on laparoscopy as it can also mimic other diagnoses such as PID. As such, a watch and wait policy is often adopted to avoid unnecessary surgery, however if the symptoms progress or the appendix has ruptured surgical intervention is required urgently.

2 a *(1 mark for each correct answer, maximum 3 marks)*   /3
   Female *(1 mark)*
   Obesity *(1 mark)*
   Age over 40 years *(1 mark)*
   Haemolytic anaemia *(1 mark)*
   Crohn's disease *(1 mark)*
   Hyperlipidaemia *(1 mark)*

b Cholesterol *(1 mark)*   /2
   Bile breakdown products *(1 mark)*

c Biliary colic *(1 mark)*   /1

d 90% are radiolucent (do not show up on x-ray),   /1
   unlike renal calculi where 90% are radio-opaque
   (do show up on x-ray) *(1 mark)*

e *(1 mark for each correct answer, maximum 2 marks)*   /2
   USS abdomen gallbladder and biliary tree *(1 mark)*
   LFTs *(1 mark)*
   FBC *(1 mark)*
   CRP *(1 mark)*
   U+E *(1 mark)*

f *(1 mark for each correct answer, maximum 3 marks)*   /3
   Gallbladder empyema *(1 mark)*
   Biliary peritonitis *(1 mark)*
   Mucocele *(1 mark)*
   Carcinoma of the gallbladder *(1 mark)*
   Obstructive jaundice *(1 mark)*
   Pancreatitis *(1 mark)*
   Cholangitis *(1 mark)*
   Gallstone ileus *(1 mark)*

Summary

The majority of gallstones are asymptomatic within the gallbladder. Their composition is of cholesterol, sometimes with breakdown products of bilirubin. In haemolytic anaemia, where there is a lot of bilirubin around, pure pigment stones can be seen. Risk factors for forming gallstones are being female, overweight, over the age of 40, having haemolytic anaemia, hyperlipidaemia and Crohn's disease.

3 a This is elicited by pressing on the RUQ and costal $\boxed{/2}$
margin *(1 mark)*. The patient is asked to take a
breath in. A positive test is when the patient
gasps in pain as the examiner's hand presses
down on an inflamed gallbladder *(1 mark)*.
For confirmation, the test should be performed
on the contralateral side and found to be negative.

b *(1 mark for each correct answer, maximum 2 marks)* $\boxed{/2}$
FBC – raised white cell count *(1 mark)*
U+E – dehydration *(1 mark)*
LFT – deranged *(1 mark)*
Amylase – acute pancreatitis may be a differential
   diagnosis *(1 mark)*
USS – confirms gallstones, thickening and oedema
   of gallbladder wall *(1 mark)*

c *(1 mark for each correct answer, maximum 2 marks)* $\boxed{/2}$
IV fluids *(1 mark)*
Antibiotics (metronidazole and augmentin) *(1 mark)*
Analgesia *(1 mark)*

d Cholecystectomy *(1 mark)* $\boxed{/1}$

e *(1 mark for each correct answer, maximum 2 marks)* $\boxed{/2}$
Less postoperative pain *(1 mark)*
A smaller wound which heals more quickly *(1 mark)*
Less chance of infection *(1 mark)*
Shorter recovery time for patient *(1 mark)*

f ERCP *(1 mark)* $\boxed{/1}$

g A remaining stone in the CBD can lead to $\boxed{/2}$
obstructive jaundice *(1 mark)*, whereby the bile
cannot escape into the duodenum as the stone
is blocking its passage *(1 mark)*

Summary

Gallstones can cause a lot of pain to the patient and can cause pancreatitis by blocking one of the pancreatic ducts at the ampulla of Vater. If the gallstone manages to pass into the duodenum without becoming obstructed it can obstruct further down at the ileocaecal valve, causing gallstone ileus. Presentation for these complications may be at a later date if the stone is not removed.

4 a They are dilated, tortuous veins *(1 mark)* $\boxed{/1}$

b *(1 mark for each correct answer, maximum 3 marks)* $\boxed{/3}$

Female *(1 mark)*
Pregnancy *(1 mark)*
Family history *(1 mark)*
Pelvic or abdominal mass *(1 mark)*
Previous DVT *(1 mark)*

c *(1 mark for each correct answer, maximum 2 marks)* `/2`
There are two systems of veins, the deep system
(which is under higher pressure) and the
superficial system *(1 mark)*. There are valves
where these two systems communicate to
prevent backflow of blood from deep to
superficial system *(1 mark)*. When these valves
don't function the pressure increases in the
superficial system and these veins swell *(1 mark)*

d *(1 mark for each correct answer, maximum 2 marks)* `/2`
The long saphenous femoral junction in the
groin *(1 mark)*
At the short saphenous popliteal vein junction
in the popliteal fossa behind the knee *(1 mark)*
Perforating veins (found in the medical side
of the calf) *(1 mark)*

e *(1 mark for each correct answer, maximum 3 marks)* `/3`
Leg ulcers (usually above the medical malleolus
where calf perforators arise) *(1 mark)*
Lipodermatosclerosis *(1 mark)*
Ankle swelling *(1 mark)*
Increased skin pigmentation (haemosiderin
deposition) *(1 mark)*
Varicose eczema *(1 mark)*

f *(1 mark for each correct answer, maximum 2 marks)* `/2`
Elevate legs where possible (this will reduce the
swelling and ease the discomfort) *(1 mark)*
Graduated compression stockings (aids venous
return of blood) *(1 mark)*
Injection sclerotherapy (small varicose veins
can be injected with a chemical that damages
the vein walls. As a result, scar tissue forms
which closes off the affected vein. Other
stronger veins take over and the treated vein,
which is no longer filled with blood, becomes
less visible) *(1 mark)*
Ligation and stripping *(1 mark)*

g Does she plan on having more children? If so a
procedure is better to be postponed until her
childbearing is finished as there is a risk of
recurrence *(1 mark)*

/1

Summary

The changes mentioned in part (e) in the legs of patients with varicose veins are only seen when the varicosities are of long standing. If a patient has significant skin changes then this is indicative
of calf perforator disease. Calf perforators are on the medial side
of the calf above the medial malleolus which is where the skin
changes are mainly seen.

5 a Intermittent claudication *(1 mark)*

/1

b *(1 mark for each correct answer, maximum 3 marks)*

/3

Smoking *(1 mark)*
Diabetes mellitus *(1 mark)*
Family history *(1 mark)*
Hyperlipidaemia *(1 mark)*
Cardiovascular disease *(1 mark)*

c *(1 mark for each correct answer, maximum 2 marks)*

/2

Stop smoking *(1 mark)*
Increase exercise tolerance (increases formation
of collateral vessels, improving blood supply to
the muscles) *(1 mark)*
Lose weight *(1 mark)*
Co-existing medical problems such as anaemia,
hyperlipidaemia, hypertension, heart failure
should be corrected *(1 mark)*
Start aspirin and statin *(1 mark)*

d *(1 mark for each correct answer, maximum 2 marks)*

/2

There is no gravity to aid blood supply to the
foot *(1 mark)*
Cardiac output drops when we sleep *(1 mark)*
The heat in bed causes vasodilatation, diverting
blood from soft tissues *(1 mark)*

e ECG (heart disease may have worsened if his
PVD has) *(1 mark)*

/3

ABPI (defines extent of ischaemia and is
a useful baseline to compare to at a later date)
(1 mark)

Angiogram (to see where the stenosis is in the
leg and to see if it is amenable to angioplasty,
which may be performed at the same time)
(1 mark)

f *(1 mark for each correct answer, maximum*
3 marks) /3

Gabapentin for pain *(1 mark)*
Balloon angioplasty *(1 mark)*
Femoral-popliteal bypass graft *(1 mark)*
Amputation *(1 mark)*

Summary

On examining a patient lying down, with arterial disease of the
leg, the leg may appear to be white if held elevated. This is due
to poor blood supply perfusing the extremity. If the leg is held
dependant on the couch, then after a minute or two the extremity
will turn bright red; this is called reactive hyperaemia. It is caused
by vasodilatation by the products of anaerobic metabolism whilst
the leg is held elevated. This is the principle of Beurger's test.

6 a Natal cleft *(1 mark)* /1
   b Can be caused by blocked ingrown hair
   follicle *(1 mark)* /1
   c *(1 mark for each correct answer, maximum 2 marks)* /2
   Staphylococcus aureus (1 mark)
   Coliform bacteria *(1 mark)*
   Gram-negative bacteria *(1 mark)*
   d Male *(1 mark)* /2
   Hirsute *(1 mark)*
   e i) Incision and drainage *(1 mark)* /2
   ii) Excision of the pilonidal sinus *(1 mark)*
   f 20% *(1 mark)* /1
   g Primary intention *(1 mark)* and secondary
   intention *(1 mark)* /2

Summary

A pilonidal sinus occurs when ingrown hairs have worked their
way under the skin. Pressure around the buttocks inhibits the body
from rejecting the hair and thus allows it to continue to burrow
deeper, which can then become infected. This condition is more
common in those whose occupation involves prolonged sitting.

7 a A direct inguinal hernia will arise medially to the $\boxed{/2}$
inferior epigastric vessels *(1 mark)*, whereas an
indirect inguinal hernia arises laterally to the
inferior epigastric vessels *(1 mark)*

b Increased abdominal pressure, e.g. heavy lifting, $\boxed{/2}$
chronic cough, obesity, straining to pass urine
(prostatism), chronic constipation (straining to
pass faeces) *(1 mark)*
Abdominal wall weakness, e.g. patent processus
vaginalis, malnutrition, advancing age, previous
surgery *(1 mark)*

c Anterior – external oblique aponeurosis *(1 mark)* $\boxed{/4}$
Posterior – transversalis fascia *(1 mark)*
Superior – conjoint tendon *(1 mark)*
Inferior – inguinal ligament *(1 mark)*

d *(1 mark for each correct answer, maximum 2 marks)* $\boxed{/2}$
Urinary retention *(1 mark)*
Ischaemic orchitis *(1 mark)*
Recurrent hernias *(1 mark)*
Scrotal haematoma *(1 mark)*
Problems with anaesthetic *(1 mark)*
Damage to ilioinguinal nerve *(1 mark)*

e *(1 mark for each correct answer, maximum 3 marks)* $\boxed{/3}$
Inguinal lymph nodes *(1 mark)*
Saphena varix (a dilated varicose vein at the
sapheno-femoral junction) *(1 mark)*
Femoral artery aneurysm *(1 mark)*
Hydrocele of the spermatic cord *(1 mark)*
Lipoma of the cord *(1 mark)*
Maldescended testicle *(1 mark)*

f This is when the neck of the hernia is very small $\boxed{/1}$
and the blood supply to the hernial contents is
impaired *(1 mark)*

Summary

A common exam question is on the differences between a femoral and an inguinal hernia. The femoral hernia emerges through the femoral canal which is below and lateral to the pubic tubercle, whereas the inguinal hernia emerges above and medial to the pubic tubercle. If a femoral hernia is diagnosed then it should be repaired as these have a higher risk of strangulation, compared to inguinal hernias which can be observed.

8 a *(1 mark for each correct answer, maximum 4 marks)* |4|
Change to bowel habit recently? *(1 mark)*
Passing any flatus? *(1 mark)*
Any contacts with similar symptoms? *(1 mark)*
Rectal bleeding? *(1 mark)*
Recent foreign travel? *(1 mark)*
Abdominal distension? *(1 mark)*
Loss of weight? *(1 mark)*
Constant or intermittent pain? *(1 mark)*
Where in the abdomen is the pain? *(1 mark)*

b To see if she had a perforated bowel which |1|
would show on a CXR as air under the
diaphragm *(1 mark)*

c *(1 mark for each correct answer, maximum 3 marks)* |3|
Tumour *(1 mark)*
Hernia *(1 mark)*
Volvulus *(1 mark)*
Diverticular disease *(1 mark)*
Faecal impaction *(1 mark)*
Stricture *(1 mark)*
Pelvic adhesions *(1 mark)*

d *(1 mark for each correct answer, maximum 4 marks)* |4|
Dukes staging *(1 mark)*
A – confined to bowel wall *(1 mark)*
B – through bowel wall *(1 mark)*
C – regional lymph node metastases *(1 mark)*
D – distant metastases (this was added later on)
  (1 mark)

e *(1 mark for each correct answer, maximum 2 marks)* |2|
High-fat, low-fibre diet *(1 mark)*
Genetic abnormalities (p53 mutations) *(1 mark)*
Inflammatory bowel disease *(1 mark)*
Family history of HNPCC or FAP or a first-degree
  relative affected *(1 mark)*

Summary

Presentation of colorectal cancer depends on the site of the tumour within the colon. Tumours on the right side are more insidious and they tend to present later with a mass or anaemia. Tumours on the left side are more likely to present with an obstruction because the faeces is more solid here and the tumour obstructs its passage.

Patients with tumours on the left present earlier with a change in bowel habit.

9 a Seminoma *(½ mark)* /1
Teratoma *(½ mark)*
 b If you can get above the lump (you should be able to /2
if it is a testicular lump but not a hernia) *(1 mark)*
Is the lump within the testis or is it separate
(lipoma of the cord) or transilluminate
(hydrocele) *(1 mark)*
 c *(1 mark for each correct answer, maximum 2 marks)* /2
The other testicle (2% are bilateral) *(1 mark)*
Abdomen for organomegaly *(1 mark)*
Lymph nodes: supraclavicular *(1 mark)*
Signs of anaemia *(1 mark)*
 d *(1 mark for each correct answer, maximum 2 marks)* /2
Serum alpha fetoprotein *(1 mark)*
Beta HCG *(1 mark)*
Placental alkaline phosphatase *(1 mark)*
FBC *(1 mark)*
U+E *(1 mark)*
 e *(1 mark for each correct answer, maximum 4 marks)* /4
Prosthetic testicle *(1 mark)*
Radiotherapy or chemotherapy (seminomas are
highly radiosensitive; teratomas are not, they
respond better to chemotherapy) *(1 mark)*
Counselling *(1 mark)*
Reassurance – prognosis is good (96–100% 5-year
survival), the tumour is confined to the testis and
has not spread *(1 mark)*
Follow-up: repeat CT scanning and tumour
markers *(1 mark)*

Summary

Germ call tumours are divided into teratomas and seminomas and mixed. A small minority of men will have bilateral tumours so a proper examination of both testicles is important. Seminomas grow slowly and metastasise to regional and para-aortic lymph nodes. Their growth is initiated in the epithelium of the seminiferous tubules. On examination it is important to check for evidence of lymphatic spread.

10 a Epididymo-orchitis *(1 mark)* `/2`
UTI *(1 mark)*
   b Urine dip and MSU for suspected UTI *(1 mark)* `/3`
Epididymo-orchitis has a longer history of
      pain and is accompanied by burning on
      voiding *(1 mark)*
O/E – with a torsion the testis lies horizontally
      or can be retracted compared to the other side
      (1 mark)
   c *(maximum 1 mark)* `/1`
If there is in fact a torsion then the blood flow
      to the testis will be compromised *(1 mark)*.
      The testis can be infarcted if the suspicion is
      not acted on and the testis lost within a few
      hours *(1 mark)*
   d That if the testicle has become infarcted then `/1`
      it must be removed at the same time
      (orchidectomy) *(1 mark)*
The other testicle will be fixed in the scrotum
      (orchidopexy) *(1 mark)*
   e Undescended testis *(1 mark)* `/1`
   f *(1 mark for each correct answer, maximum 3 marks)* `/3`
An enlarged scrotum *(1 mark)*
Tenderness *(1 mark)*
Redness *(1 mark)*
Pain on micturition *(1 mark)*
Penile discharge *(1 mark)*
Fever *(1 mark)*
   g *(1 mark for each correct answer, maximum 2 marks)* `/2`
STI *(1 mark)*
UTI (bacteria from a UTI can track back down
      to the vas deferens) *(1 mark)*
Mumps *(1 mark)*
Complication of post-prostatectomy *(1 mark)*

Summary

Testicular torsion is most common between the ages of 12 and
27 years. It presents with sudden onset of severe pain that is constant in nature. If this diagnosis is in question the patient is taken
for an exploration in theatre. If this is not done the testicle can
infarct and is lost, decreasing fertility. In theatre both testicles

are fixed with a suture to the scrotal wall to prevent torsion in future.

11 a Fibroadenoma *(1 mark)* /3
   Carcinoma *(1 mark)*
   Breast cyst *(1 mark)*
  b *(1 mark for each correct answer, maximum 4 marks)* /4
   Recently given birth? *(1 mark)*
   Nipple discharge? *(1 mark)*
   Nipple inversion? *(1 mark)*
   Family history of breast cancer? *(1 mark)*
   On OCP? *(1 mark)*
   Has she noticed if lump has increased in size?
      (1 mark)
  c Fibroadenoma *(1 mark)* /1
  d *(1 mark for each correct answer, maximum 2 marks)* /2
   Mammogram *(1 mark)*
   USS *(1 mark)*
   Tru-cut biopsy *(1 mark)*
  e Nothing specific. Advise her to return to her /1
   GP if the lump increases in size or becomes
   painful *(1 mark)*
  f No *(1 mark)* /1

Summary

Fibroadenoma is most common before the age of 30. Collagenous mesenchyme within the breast proliferates under the influence of oestrogen and progesterone. Patients tend to present young, with a mobile firm breast lump, which can be left and observed or excised. Occasionally they can grow to be very large but this is rare. They are benign and do not increase the risk of cancer, although they can be very worrying for the patient.

12 a *(1 mark for each correct answer, maximum 4 marks)* /4
   Has she reached menopause? *(1 mark)*
   Nulliparous *(1 mark)*
   Older age of having first child *(1 mark)*
   Early menarche *(1 mark)*
   Family history of breast or ovarian cancer *(1 mark)*
   Obese *(1 mark)*
   Use of exogenous oestrogens *(1 mark)*

Surface erythema *(1 mark)*

Ulceration *(1 mark)*

Change in size of breast *(1 mark)*

Previous problems with breasts, cysts etc.
and how long ago

b *(1 mark for each correct answer, maximum 2 marks)* /2

Sentinel node biopsy *(1 mark)*

Stage and grade the tumour *(1 mark)*

Is it herceptin and oestrogen receptor positive?
(1 mark)

c *(1 mark for each correct answer, maximum 2 marks)* /2

The stage of a cancer describes its size and
whether it has spread beyond its original site
(1 mark). Grading refers to the appearance of
the cancer cells under the microscope *(1 mark)*.
The grade gives an idea of how quickly the
cancer may develop *(1 mark)*

d Hormonal therapies such as tamoxifen and /3
herceptin *(1 mark)*

Chemotherapy *(1 mark)*

Radiotherapy *(1 mark)*

e *(1 mark for each correct answer, maximum* /2
2 marks)

Liver *(1 mark)*

Brain *(1 mark)*

Lungs *(1 mark)*

Bone marrow *(1 mark)*

Bone *(1 mark)*

Summary

The disturbance to a woman's body image after a mastectomy can be devastating, with some women chosing to have reconstructive surgery, although increasingly surgeons are able to offer reconstructive surgery to minimise asymmetry at the time of resection. There are a couple of options as regards implants. One option is a bag of silicone surrounded by an outer sheath which can be inflated with saline. This is placed under the pectoralis major muscle. The other option is a myocutaneous flap which can be taken from latissimus dorsi or from the lower part of the rectus abdominis muscle.

13 a *(1 mark for each correct answer, maximum 4 marks)* 　　/4

Re-dip her urine *(1 mark)*

MSU *(1 mark)*

Bloods: FBC, CRP, U+E, glucose, blood cultures
(maximum 1 mark)

Renal USS *(1 mark)*

BM *(1 mark)*

b *(1 mark for each correct answer, maximum 4 marks)* 　　/4

NBM *(1 mark)*

Admit *(1 mark)*

Cannulate and IV fluids *(1 mark)*

Analgesia and anti-emetic *(1 mark)*

IV antibiotics *(1 mark)*

Monitor BMs (often high during concurrent
illness) and treat accordingly *(1 mark)*

Refer to urology *(1 mark)*

c *(1 mark for each correct answer, maximum 2 marks)* 　　/2

Re-dip urine to check infection has cleared
(1 mark)

Urology outpatient appointment after discharge
(1 mark)

Imaging to check kidney *(1 mark)*

d *(1 mark for each correct answer, maximum 2 marks)* 　　/2

Diabetes mellitus *(1 mark)*

Female gender (the female urethra is longer than
the male urethra, and because the urinary
meatus is in close proximity to the vagina
bacteria can easily spread from the vagina up
the urinary tract) *(1 mark)*

Vesicoureteral reflux *(1 mark)*

Pregnancy *(1 mark)*

Long-term indwelling catheter *(1 mark)*

Summary

Patients with pyelonephritis, especially the elderly, can become septic quickly. Signs to look for are low BP and a high pulse rate (which can indicate shock), temperature >40°C and new onset of renal impairment. Elderly patients may not be febrile but can still be heavily bacteraemic. Urgent treatment is required as scarring of the renal tract including the kidneys can occur and may lead to chronic renal failure.

14 a *(1 mark for each correct answer, maximum 3 marks)* /3

FBC (WCC >15) *(1 mark)*

U+E (urea >16) *(1 mark)*

Amylase (usually >1000 but may be normal if chronic pancreatitis) *(1 mark)*

CRP (raised) *(1 mark)*

LFT (albumin <32) *(1 mark)*

Calcium levels (<2.0) *(1 mark)*

LDH (>300 IU/L) *(1 mark)*

Glucose (>11.1 mmol) *(1 mark)*

Arterial blood gases (pO_2 <8.1) *(1 mark)*

AXR – looking for a 'sentinel loop' where the proximal jejunum becomes dilated. Also gas and fluid levels may be seen *(1 mark)*

CXR – ARDS and pleural effusion *(1 mark)*

b *(1 mark for each correct answer, maximum 4 marks)* /4

Gallstones *(1 mark)*

Alcohol *(1 mark)*

Idiopathic *(1 mark)*

Trauma *(1 mark)*

Tumours of pancreas and biliary tree *(1 mark)*

Steroids *(1 mark)*

Mumps *(1 mark)*

Autoimmune disease *(1 mark)*

Hyperlipidaemia *(1 mark)*

Hypercalcaemia *(1 mark)*

ERCP *(1 mark)*

Scorpion bite *(1 mark)*

Drugs e.g. Azathiporine *(1 mark)*

c *(1 mark for each correct answer, maximum 3 marks)* /3

IV fluids *(1 mark)*

Insert a urinary catheter and measure output hourly – output should be at least 30 ml each hour *(1 mark)*

Analgesia and antiemetic *(1 mark)*

NBM *(1 mark)*

Try to find cause – USS for gallstones *(1 mark)*

Call for senior help *(1 mark)*

d Early – ARDS, shock, acute renal failure, DIC, hypocalcaemia (enzymes are released from the pancreas which binds to calcium, taking it out of circulation), hyperglycaemia (islet cells which produce insulin are destroyed) *(1 mark each, maximum 2 marks)* /4

Late – pseudocyst (a collection in the lesser sac),
haemorrhage, necrosis of bowel, chronic pain,
pancreatic insufficiency (creon needed to prevent
symptoms such as steatorrhoea, weight loss),
diabetes mellitus, chronic pancreatitis, recurrence
(1 mark each, maximum 2 marks)

Summary

Patients with acute pancreatitis present with severe epigastric
pain radiating to the back. Patients with this condition can deteriorate rapidly, and so prompt treatment with IV fluids and analgesia should be instigated. A measure of severity of pancreatitis is
Modified Glasgow Criteria. These should all be measured within
48 hours of admission. More than 3 suggests severe pancreatitis. The
criteria fit neatly into the mnemonic PANCREAS. These are: PO_2
<8 kPa, Age >55 years, Neutrophils: WCC >15, Calcium <2 mmol,
Renal function: urea >16 mmol/L, Enzymes: LDH >600 IU/L, AST
>200 IU/L, Albumin <32 g/L, Sugar: blood glucose >10 mmol/L.

15 a *(1 mark for each correct answer, maximum 3 marks)* ☐ /3
   Venous ulcer *(1 mark)*
   Arterial ulcer *(1 mark)*
   Neuropathic ulcer *(1 mark)*
   Decubitus ulcer (pressure sore) *(1 mark)*
 b *(1 mark for each correct answer, maximum 3 marks)* ☐ /3
   Venous ulcer – lower leg, venous eczema, painful,
     brown pigmentation from haemosiderin, varicose
     veins, lipodermatosclerosis, atrophie blanche
     (1 mark for 2 features)
   Arterial ulcer – punched out, painful, higher up
     on legs or feet, may give history of claudication
     (1 mark for 2 features)
   Neuropathic ulcer – seen over pressure areas,
     diabetics, no sensation *(1 mark for 2 features)*
   Decubitus ulcer – occur in elderly, immobile
     patients, due to skin ischaemia over bony
     prominence *(1 mark for 2 features)*
 c HbA1c to assess adherence to diet and ☐ /2
     medication *(1 mark)*
   US studies to assess for any additional underlying
     arterial or venous disease *(1 mark)*

d Intermittent claudication *(1 mark)*   ☐ /2
Leriche syndrome *(1 mark)*

e There are incompetent valves in the deep or   ☐ /2
perforating veins *(1 mark)* which allows sustained
venous hypertension in superficial veins *(1 mark)*
to develop and varicosities to form.

Summary

Venous ulceration is usually found above the medial malleolus. This is where the calf perforator veins arise. The majority of leg ulcers are venous in origin. Arterial ulcers are situated anywhere on the leg or foot, depending on where the occlusion is. Arterial ulcers can be accompanied by other signs of PVD such as gangrene, which usually occurs in the peripheries, e.g. the toes.

16 a Outpouching of mucosa through weak areas   ☐ /2
near blood vessels in the muscle wall *(1 mark)*
due to high intraluminal pressures *(1 mark)*

b *(1 mark for each correct answer, maximum 2 marks)*   ☐ /2
Low-fibre diet *(1 mark)*
Constipation which causes increased intra-colonic
  pressure causing herniation *(1 mark)*
Old age *(1 mark)*
Following a western diet *(1 mark)*

c *(1 mark for each correct answer, maximum 2 marks)*   ☐ /2
NBM, IV fluids, NG tube (gut rest) *(1 mark)*
Bloods – clotting, FBC, U+E, CRP *(1 mark)*
AXR/CT abdomen – imaging *(1 mark)*
Antibiotics (augmentin and metronidazole) *(1 mark)*
Surgery if symptoms worsen *(1 mark)*

d *(maximum 1 mark)*   ☐ /1
Erythromycin *(½ mark)*
Ciprofloxacin *(½ mark)*
Teicoplanin *(½ mark)*

e *(1 mark for each correct answer, maximum 5 marks)*   ☐ /5
Inflammatory bowel syndrome *(1 mark)*
Pelvic floor dyssynergia *(1 mark)*
Intestinal obstruction *(1 mark)*
Pseudo-obstruction *(1 mark)*
Painful anal conditions *(1 mark)*
Drugs: opiates, aluminium antacids *(1 mark)*

Hypothyroidism, hypercalcaemia *(1 mark)*
Spinal cord lesion *(1 mark)*
Depression *(1 mark)*
Immobility *(1 mark)*
Hirshsprung's *(1 mark)*

Summary

Diverticular disease commonly occurs in the sigmoid colon and is a common finding in about half of people over 50 years of age and is usually asymptomatic in 95% of them. In flare-ups, with simple gut rest, fluids and antibiotics the majority settle and are able to be discharged home.

17 a *(1 mark for each correct answer, maximum 4 marks)*   /4
Length of symptoms? *(1 mark)*
Medications on? e.g. ferrous sulphate turns faeces
   black *(1 mark)*
Change in bowel habit? *(1 mark)*
Has he noticed any masses in his abdomen?
   (1 mark)
Any unusual bloating? *(1 mark)*
How is his appetite? *(1 mark)*
Current eating/drinking habits? *(1 mark)*
Colour and amount of rectal bleeding? *(1 mark)*
b *(1 mark for each correct answer, maximum 2 marks)*   /2
Family history, e.g. FAP, HNPCC *(1 mark)*
Smoking *(1 mark)*
High animal fat intake *(1 mark)*
Inflammatory bowel disease *(1 mark)*
c *(1 mark for each correct answer, maximum 2 marks)*   /2
AXR *(1 mark)*
Staging CT *(1 mark)*
Double-contrast barium enema *(1 mark)*
Colonoscopy + biopsy *(1 mark)*
d *(1 mark for each correct answer, maximum 3 marks)*   /3
Prolapse *(1 mark)*
Parastomal hernia *(1 mark)*
Skin irritation at site of stoma *(1 mark)*
Ulceration *(1 mark)*
Necrosis of bowel mucosa *(1 mark)*
Psychological issue *(1 mark)*

Summary

Colon cancer typically presents with weight loss and blood in the stool. There may be an altered bowel habit or obstruction, and patient with tumours in the ascending colon often present later with these symptoms. Tumours are most common in the rectum and sigmoid colon, which can be viewed on rigid sigmoidoscopy. However, colonoscopy is required to exclude tumours elsewhere and take a biopsy. Colorectal cancer is the second most common cause of cancer death in the UK. The average age at diagnosis tends to be around 60 years; it is much more common in western countries due to a diet low in fibre.

18 a Haemorrhoids *(1 mark)* `/1`

  b *(1 mark for each correct answer, maximum 2 marks)* `/2`
    Chronic constipation *(1 mark)*
    Obesity *(1 mark)*
    Family history *(1 mark)*

  c *(1 mark for each correct answer, maximum 2 marks)* `/2`
    Pruritus ani *(1 mark)*
    Perianal swelling *(1 mark)*
    Perianal discomfort *(1 mark)*
    Prolapse *(1 mark)*

  d First degree – small, don't prolapse *(1 mark)* `/3`
    Second degree – small and prolapsed but
      spontaneously reduce *(1 mark)*
    Third degree – prolapsing haemorrhoids which
      require manual reduction *(1 mark)*

  e *(1 mark for each correct answer, maximum 4 marks)* `/4`
    Creams – symptomatic relief *(1 mark)*
    Injection sclerotherapy *(1 mark)*
    Banding *(1 mark)*
    Cryotherapy *(1 mark)*
    Haemorroidectomy *(1 mark)*

Summary

A haemorrhoid is an anal cushion which drains into the superior rectal vein. Haemorrhoids occur when rectal pressure is high, e.g. constipation or pregnancy. Patients will typically present with bright red blood around the outside of the stool and on wiping. On examining a patient haemorrhoids will be seen in the 3, 7 and 11 o'clock positions and a rectal examination is necessary to exclude a rectal tumour, as many patients will be concerned about this.

Practice Paper 1

QUESTIONS

1 Maria, a 42-year-old lady, has been diagnosed with hyperthyroidism.

   a Give three clinical signs of hyperthyroidism.   *3 marks*
   b Give two medical treatments for this condition.   *2 marks*
   c What is the role of the thyroid gland?   *2 marks*
   d She opts for a total thyroidectomy. What further treatment will she need to be on after the operation?   *1 mark*
   e Postoperatively her calcium level comes back at 1.78 (2.00–2.40). What is the cause of this?   *1 mark*
   f Name one special sign you may be able to elicit.   *1 mark*
   g Explain the fundamental aspects of calcium homeostasis.   *3 marks*

2 A 35-year-old woman comes to see you in clinic after experiencing post-coital bleeding on and off for the last 7–8 months. She has become aware of a fullness in her abdomen.

   a What three further questions might you ask to confirm or refute a diagnosis?   *3 marks*
   b What three investigations would you order?   *3 marks*
   c A large fibroid is found in her uterus. Give three treatment options.   *3 marks*
   d How are the findings on a cervical smear graded?   *2 marks*
   e Name the virus, and the particular strains, believed to give rise to cervical cancer.   *1 mark*
   f Name two risk factors for cervical cancer.   *2 marks*

3 Sophie, a 35-year-old recent divorcee, presents to you feeling low in mood for a couple of weeks, and reports that she doesn't want to live any more because she is getting a message to die

Complete SAQs for Medical Finals By P. Stather et al, Published 2010 by Blackwell Publishing, ISBN: 978-1-4501-8928-6.

from an orbiting satellite. When you confront her regarding this she is adamant that this is happening and becomes annoyed.

a Identify three biological symptoms of depression. *3 marks*

b Give three different types of antidepressants available and give an example of each. *3 marks*

c What is a delusion? *2 marks*

d Give six risk factors for suicide. *3 marks*

e Name three common Sections of the Mental Health Act used to detain patients. *3 marks*

4 Iqbal, a 76-year-old diabetic male, has had chronic renal failure for a number of years. During a routine appointment a blood test was performed which revealed a potassium level of 6.7 mmol/L.

a What is the definition of chronic renal failure? *1 mark*

b Name six signs and symptoms you would look for in a patient with chronic renal failure. *3 marks*

c Other than diabetes, give two causes of chronic renal failure. *2 marks*

d What changes would you look for on an ECG in a patient with hyperkalaemia? *2 marks*

e Give four causes of hyperkalaemia. *2 marks*

f How would you treat hyperkalaemia? *3 marks*

g The patient unfortunately develops VT; name an ECG feature of VT. How is VT treated? *2 marks*

5 Samuel is a 68-year-old gentleman referred to the ophthalmology clinic by his GP after complaining of patchy visual loss. He is an insulin-dependent diabetic who also has hypertension and hypercholesterolaemia. You suspect this to be a case of retinopathy.

a Give two alternative diagnoses. *2 marks*

b What are the first four classes of diabetic retinopathy? *4 marks*

c What other organs are likely to be affected in this patient? *1 mark*

d What agencies/other disciplines may need to be initiated in supporting Samuel as his vision deteriorates? Name three. *3 marks*

e Identify three broad steps you might take in the management of Samuel's condition. *3 marks*

f Explain how sulphonylureas (e.g. gliclazide) work. *2 marks*

g Give two common side effects of metformin. *2 marks*

6 Simon, a 7-year-old boy, suffers from cystic fibrosis. He has now become unwell with an increasingly productive cough, fever, tachycardia and worsening tachypnoea.

   a Name three 'bedside' tests you would perform.   *3 marks*

   b What does spirometry measure?   *2 marks*

   c He also looks malnourished and small for his age. How can you assess this?   *1 mark*

   d Why is he malnourished?   *2 marks*

   e He subsequently made a good recovery and was discharged. Several months later he developed similar symptoms but this time a CXR showed a small pleural effusion. What three signs will you try to elicit on clinical examination?   *3 marks*

   f You perform a diagnostic pleural aspiration. Where in relation to the rib will you insert your needle?   *2 marks*

7 An 18-year-old called Callum, who has suffered from epilepsy since childhood, has a seizure. He has had three seizures in the last 4 months, which is unusual as it is normally well controlled with phenytoin. He is admitted to hospital.

   a Name three features of your immediate management.   *3 marks*

   b Other than non-compliance with medication, give three possible causes for Callum's seizure.   *3 marks*

   c Despite your best efforts Callum has been fitting for 32 minutes. What name is given to this condition?   *1 mark*

   d When his blood results come back you find that his phenytoin level is well below the therapeutic range. When he comes around he reveals he has not been taking his phenytoin due to side-effects. Give three side-effects of phenytoin.   *3 marks*

   e By what mechanism does excess alcohol give rise to a seizure?   *1 mark*

8 Mavis is 83 and has a past medical history that includes high cholesterol, hypertension and Paget's disease. She is admitted from her nursing home following a fall. She is now unable to bear weight on her right leg and you suspect a fracture of the neck of femur.

   a Describe the pathological process that causes Paget's disease.   *2 marks*

b Give two features of Paget's disease. *2 marks*

c What is the term given to describe the characteristic features of Paget's disease seen on x-rays? *1 mark*

d What two features (other than pain) might you see on examination of a patient with a fractured neck of femur? *2 marks*

e What is the major risk of a fracture of the femoral neck and how does it occur? *2 marks*

f Mavis is treated with surgical fixation but is slow to mobilise. On her sixth day postoperatively Mavis complains of chest pain and in view of her lack of mobility you suspect a pulmonary embolism. Give three questions you will ask Mavis regarding the possibility of a clot. *3 marks*

g Mavis's sats are 88% on room air and you perform an ABG which confirms she is hypoxic. What might you see on:

  i) a chest x-ray *1 mark*

  ii) a CTPA *1 mark*

9 Abbey, a 23-year-old woman, presents to her GP complaining of recurrent diarrhoea and abdominal pain over the last 2 months. Her stools are loose with blood mixed in. She is opening her bowels 5–6 times a day and has lost 1 stone during the past 2 months which has been unintentional.

a Given this history, what three initial investigations would you want to perform? *3 marks*

b Crohn's disease is diagnosed. Name three GI complications of the disease. *3 marks*

c Abbey's Hb is low at 10.5 and her vitamin B12 levels are also low. What do these results indicate in a patient with Crohn's disease? *1 mark*

d She fails to respond to first-line therapies and although she has no serious complications her symptoms persist. What other two classes of drug could you try long term? *2 marks*

e Although these are effective drugs, name two main side-effects to each class of drug you have mentioned in part (d). *4 marks*

10 Paul, a 72-year-old diabetic man with hypertension, presents to
A & E with sudden-onset central chest pain and vomiting. His
initial investigation results suggest a NSTEMI. He is given morphine, aspirin, antiemetics and GTN, then transferred to CCU.

    a On day 6 he is very breathless and you suspect
       left ventricular failure; name six symptoms and
       signs of this.   *3 marks*

    b Name two features of left ventricular failure as
       seen on a CXR.   *2 marks*

    c Define cardiomegaly.   *1 mark*

    d Give two common causes of ventricular failure.   *2 marks*

    e Name three drugs used in the treatment of
       heart failure   *3 marks*

    f A few days later his sodium level is found to be
       125 mmol/L. Give two causes of this, and what
       investigations would you instigate?   *4 marks*

Practice Paper 1

ANSWERS

1 a *(maximum 3 marks)*   /3
   Tremor *(1 mark)*
   Palmar erythema *(1 mark)*
   Onycholysis *(1 mark)*
   Acropachy *(1 mark)*
   Exopthalmos *(1 mark)*
   Lid retraction *(1 mark)*
   Lid lag *(1 mark)*
   Goitre *(1 mark)*
   Increased sweating *(1 mark)*
   Tachycardia *(1 mark)*
   AF *(1 mark)*
   Hyper-reflexia *(1 mark)*

b *(maximum 2 marks)*   /2
   Radioactive iodine *(1 mark)*
   Carbimazole *(1 mark)*
   Propylthiouracil *(1 mark)*

c To produce T3/T4 which help to regulate growth   /2
   and metabolism *(1 mark)*

d Levothyroxine *(1 mark)*   /1

e The parathyroid glands have been removed *(1 mark)* /1

f *(maximum 1 mark)*   /1
   Chvostek's sign – tap on the facial nerve to cause
      twitching *(1 mark)*
   Trousseau's sign – inflate a BP cuff to cause tingling
      and muscular fibrillation *(1 mark)*

g *(maximum 3 marks)*   /3
   Vitamin D and parathyroid hormone (PTH)
      increase calcium absorption from the gut
      (1 mark). The kidneys work to adjust calcium
      reabsorption depending on PTH levels *(1 mark)*,
      and PTH also increases osteoclast activity to absorb
      calcium into the bones *(1 mark)*

2 a *(maximum 3 marks)* `/3`
Regular menses? *(1 mark)*
Heavy menses? *(1 mark)*
Up to date with cervical screening? *(1 mark)*
Change in sexual partner 7–8 months ago? *(1 mark)*
Intermenstrual bleeding? *(1 mark)*
Bowel and bladder symptoms? *(1 mark)*
Any children of her own? *(1 mark)*

b *(maximum 3 marks)* `/3`
FBC – looking for anaemia *(1 mark)*
Triple swabs – looking for STIs *(1 mark)*
Cervical smear – cervical cancer? *(1 mark)*
US abdomen – can show endometrial thickening
    (1 mark)
Transvaginal ultrasound *(1 mark)*

c Myomectomy *(1 mark)* `/3`
Uterine artery embolisation *(1 mark)*
Hysterectomy *(1 mark)*

d CIN 1 = mild dyskaryosis `/2`
CIN 2 = moderate dyskaryosis
CIN 3 = severe dyskaryosis
(½ mark each, 2 marks if all correct)

e Human papillomas virus strains 16 and 18 `/1`
    (½ mark each)

f *(maximum 2 marks)* `/2`
Multiple sexual partners *(1 mark)*
Early age at first sexual intercourse *(1 mark)*
Smoking *(1 mark)*
Increasing age *(1 mark)*

3 a *(maximum 3 marks)* `/3`
Sleep disturbance *(1 mark)*
Loss of appetite *(1 mark)*
Weight loss *(1 mark)*
Constipation *(1 mark)*
Loss of libido *(1 mark)*
Amenorrhoea *(1 mark)*

b *(maximum 3 marks)* `/3`
Tricyclic antidepressants – amitriptyline, dosulepin
    (1 mark)
Monoamine oxidase inhibitors – phenelzine,
    isocarboxazid *(1 mark)*

Selective serotonin reuptake inhibitors – fluoxetine, citalopram, paroxetine, sertraline *(1 mark)*

Serotonin noradrenaline reuptake inhibitor – venlafaxine, duloxetine *(1 mark)*

c A false, firm, unshakeable and fixed belief *(1 mark)* which is not in keeping with the individual's social, cultural and religious background *(1 mark)*

`/2`

d *(maximum 3 marks)*

`/3`

Hopelessness *(½ mark)*

Previous suicide attempt *(½ mark)*

Major life event *(½ mark)*

Social isolation *(½ mark)*

Older age *(½ mark)*

Depressive disorder *(½ mark)*

Alcohol *(½ mark)*

Drug use *(½ mark)*

Schizophrenia *(½ mark)*

Chronic illness *(½ mark)*

Epilepsy *(½ mark)*

Personality disorder *(½ mark)*

Male gender *(½ mark)*

Unemployment *(½ mark)*

e Section 5.2 – Doctors holding power with a duration of up to 72 hours *(1 mark)*

`/3`

Section 2 – Authority to detain an individual in hospital for assessment for up to 28 days *(1 mark)*

Section 3 – Authority to detain an individual in hospital for treatment for up to 6 months *(1 mark)*

4 a A long-standing, gradually progressive and substantial decrease in renal function *(1 mark)*

`/1`

b *(maximum 3 marks)*

`/3`

Bruising *(½ mark)*

Pallor *(½ mark)*

Brown nails *(½ mark)*

Jaundice *(½ mark)*

Excoriation *(½ mark)*

Hypertension *(½ mark)*

Oedema *(½ mark)*

Myopathy *(½ mark)*

Neuropathy *(½ mark)*

Pericarditis *(½ mark)*
Effusions *(½ mark)*

c *(maximum 2 marks)* `/2`
Hypertension *(1 mark)*
Glomerulonephritis *(1 mark)*
Obstructive uropathy *(1 mark)*
Interstitial nephritis *(1 mark)*

d *(maximum 2 marks)* `/2`
Tall tented T waves *(1 mark)*
Wide QRS complex *(1 mark)*
Flat P waves *(1 mark)*

e *(maximum 2 marks)* `/2`
Renal failure *(½ mark)*
Iatrogenic – potassium-sparing diuretics *(½ mark)*,
    ACE inhibitors *(½ mark)*, potassium therapy *(½ mark)*
Burns *(½ mark)*
Diabetic ketoacidosis *(½ mark)*
Addison's disease *(½ mark)*
Large blood transfusion *(½ mark)*

f *(maximum 3 marks)* `/3`
Calcium gluconate *(1 mark)*
Insulin and dextrose infusion *(1 mark)*
Calcium resonium *(1 mark)*
Nebulised salbutamol *(1 mark)*

g Features – QRS concordancy, capture beats, `/2`
    fusion beats, wide QRS *(1 mark for 1 example)*
Treatment – electrocardioversion *(1 mark)*

5 a Cataract *(1 mark)* `/2`
Macular degeneration *(1 mark)*

b Background – microaneurysms, dot and blot `/4`
    haemorrhages, exudates *(1 mark)*
Preproliferative – cotton wool spots, venous
    bleeding, loops and doubling *(1 mark)*
Proliferative – new vessels at the disc and
    elsewhere *(1 mark)*
Maculopathy – microaneurysms, haemorrhages,
    exudates, oedema at the macula *(1 mark)*

c Kidneys *(1 mark)* `/1`

d *(maximum 3 marks)* `/3`
Occupational therapy *(1 mark)*
Social Services for benefits *(1 mark)*

Royal National Institute for the Blind *(1 mark)*
Peer support groups *(1 mark)*
Guide Dogs Association *(1 mark)*

e *(maximum 3 marks)* /3
Strict diabetic control *(1 mark)*
Strict BP control *(1 mark)*
Regular screening and outpatient follow-up *(1 mark)*
Fluorescein angiography to identify new vessels as
    targets for laser treatment *(1 mark)*

f *(maximum 2 marks)* /2
They stimulate insulin secretion *(1 mark)* by binding
to sulphonylurea receptors *(1 mark)* and blocking
potassium channels *(1 mark)* which leads to the
release of insulin. They also inhibit gluconeogenesis.
(1 mark)

g *(maximum 2 marks)* /2
Anorexia *(1 mark)*
Weight loss *(1 mark)*
Nausea and vomiting *(1 mark)*
Abdominal pain *(1 mark)*
Diarrhoea *(1 mark)*
Lactic acidosis *(1 mark)*

6 a Sputum culture *(1 mark)* /3
Peak expiratory flow rate *(1 mark)*
Oxygen saturation *(1 mark)*

b *(maximum 2 marks)* /2
FEV1 *(1 mark)*
FVC *(1 mark)*
Total lung capacity *(1 mark)*
Tidal volume *(1 mark)*

c Plot serial height and weight on a /1
centile chart *(1 mark)*

d *(maximum 2 marks)* /2
Poor absorption *(1 mark)* and poor digestion *(1 mark)*
due to reduction of pancreatic enzyme secretion
secondary to its dysfunction *(1 mark)*

e *(maximum 3 marks)* /3
Reduced expansion *(1 mark)*
Stony dull percussion *(1 mark)*
Decreased air entry *(1 mark)*
Decreased vocal resonance *(1 mark)*

f Percuss upper border of effusion and choose
a site two intercostal spaces below it *(1 mark)*.
Aim to insert needle just above the rib as the
intercostal vessels and nerves lie just below
the rib *(1 mark)*

`/2`

7 a *(maximum 3 marks)*

`/3`

Blood sugar measurement *(1 mark)*
Oxygen *(1 mark)*
Take blood for electrolytes, calcium, magnesium,
    toxicology, phenytoin levels *(1 mark)*
Monitor ECG *(1 mark)*
Cannulate *(1 mark)*
BP *(1 mark)*
Rectal diazepam if still fitting *(1 mark)*

b *(maximum 3 marks)*

`/3`

Alcohol excess *(1 mark)*
Flashing lights *(1 mark)*
Sleep deprivation *(1 mark)*
Fever *(1 mark)*
Emotional disturbances *(1 mark)*

c Status epilepticus *(1 mark)*

`/1`

d *(maximum 3 marks)*

`/3`

Gingival hypertrophy and tenderness *(1 mark)*
Cerebellar symptoms – slurred speech *(1 mark)*,
    ataxic gait *(1 mark)*, blurred vision *(1 mark)*
Peripheral neuropathy *(1 mark)*
Coarsening of facial features *(1 mark)*
Acne and hirsutism *(1 mark)*

e Hypoglycaemia *(1 mark)*.

`/1`

8 a *(maximum 2 marks)*

`/2`

There is localized excessive osteoclastic resorption
of bone *(1 mark)* which is followed by disordered
osteoblastic activity *(1 mark)* and the formation of
new bone that is weak because it is structurally
abnormal *(1 mark)*

b *(maximum 2 marks)*

`/2`

Deafness *(1 mark)*
Fractures of long bones *(1 mark)*
Optic atrophy *(1 mark)*
Hypercalcaemia *(1 mark)*

High-output cardiac failure *(1 mark)*
Osteogenic sarcoma *(1 mark)*
Osteoarthritis of related joints *(1 mark)*

c Lytic lesions *(1 mark)* `/1`

d External rotation of affected limb *(1 mark)* `/2`
Shortening of affected limb *(1 mark)*

e Avascular necrosis *(1 mark)* – it occurs due to `/2`
disruption to the blood supply to the
femoral head via the circumflex femoral
artery *(1 mark)*

f *(maximum 3 marks)* `/3`
Is the pain pleuritic (worse on inspiration)? *(1 mark)*
Does she feel short of breath? *(1 mark)*
Does she have any areas of swelling, tenderness,
   warmth on her legs? (i.e. DVT) *(1 mark)*
Does she have any other risk factors for developing
   a clot? (i.e. history of malignancy, family/personal
   history of clot) *(1 mark)*

g i) CXR – wedge-shaped shadow or atelectasis `/1`
   (1 mark)
   ii) CTPA – filling defects *(1 mark)* `/1`

9 a Blood tests including FBC, CRP, ESR and `/3`
   haematinics *(1 mark)*
   Flexible sigmoidoscopy *(1 mark)*
   Stool culture *(1 mark)*
   Small bowel barium follow-through *(1 mark)*

b Small bowel obstruction secondary to `/3`
   stricture *(1 mark)*
   Fistulae formation *(1 mark)*
   Anal fissures *(1 mark)*
   Abscesses *(1 mark)*

c Terminal ileal disease *(1 mark)* `/1`

d Immunosuppressants – azathioprine *(1 mark)* `/2`
   Biological agents – infliximab *(1 mark)*

e Immunosuppressants – hypersensitivity reactions, `/4`
   bone marrow suppression, liver impairment,
   increased susceptibility to infections *(1 mark
   per example, maximum 2 marks)*
   Biological agents – dyspepsia, hepatitis, cholecystitis,
   GI haemorrhage, flushing, bradycardia *(1 mark per
   example, maximum 2 marks)*

10 a *(maximum 3 marks)*   /3
   Fatigue (1 *mark*)
   Orthopnoea *(1 mark)*
   Paroxysmal nocturnal dyspnoea *(1 mark)*
   Cardiomegaly *(1 mark)*
   Displaced apex beat *(1 mark)*
   Pulmonary oedema *(1 mark)*
   Tachycardia *(1 mark)*
   Bibasal crepitations *(1 mark)*
   Dyspnoea *(1 mark)*
   Nocturnal cough *(1 mark)*

   b *(maximum 2 marks)*   /2
   Pulmonary oedema *(1 mark)*
   Kerley B lines *(1 mark)*
   Cardiomegaly *(1 mark)*
   Dilated upper lobe vessels *(1 mark)*
   Pleural effusion *(1 mark)*

   c Cardiothoracic ratio of greater than 50% *(1 mark)*   /1

   d *(maximum 2 marks)*   /2
   Myocardial disease (IHD, HTN) *(1 mark)*
   Volume overload *(1 mark)*
   Valvular disease *(1 mark)*
   High metabolic demand (Paget's, hyperthyroid)
      (1 mark)
   Pericardial tamponade *(1 mark)*
   Arrhythmias *(1 mark)*
   Excess alcohol consumption *(1 mark)*

   e *(maximum 3 marks)*   /3
   Loop diuretics *(1 mark)*
   ACE inhibitors *(1 mark)*
   Beta-blocker *(1 mark)*
   Spironolactone *(1 mark)*
   Nitrates *(1 mark)*
   Calcium channel blockers *(1 mark)*

   f Causes: iatrogenic, high water intake,   /4
      hypothyroidism, Addison's disease
      (1 mark per example, maximum 2 marks)
   Investigations: urine osmolality, serum
      osmolality, TFT, 9 a.m. cortisol, short
      synacthen test *(1 mark per example,
      maximum 2 marks)*

Practice Paper 2

QUESTIONS

1 You are reviewing Alex, a 69-year-old gentleman, in clinic. He is known to have angina, for which he uses his GTN spray at least once per week.

  a Explain the pathophysiology behind angina.   *2 marks*

  b When does the heart receive its blood supply during the cardiac cycle?   *1 mark*

  c When the heart rate doubles, what happens to the coronary artery filling time?   *1 mark*

  d Explain two ways in which GTN works.   *2 marks*

  e What medication may you use to decrease Alex's use of GTN?   *1 mark*

  f He later presents to A & E with chest pain which has not been relieved by his GTN. He also looks pale and sweaty, and is in considerable discomfort. Which four medications should the ambulance team have given him?   *4 marks*

  g You perform an ECG which shows ST elevation in leads V4–V6. Where is the location of his infarct?   *1 mark*

  h What two options are there to treat this?   *2 marks*

2 Barry, a 58-year-old diabetic, presents with a cold numb right foot and a large ulcer above the ankle. He has a significant past history of an MI and CABG, which is not helped by his weight of 120 kg with a height of 1.7 m.

  a Calculate Barry's BMI.   *1 mark*

  b What is the optimum BMI range for this patient?   *1 mark*

  c Given his history, what are the two most likely types of ulcers this man may have? State two ways of distinguishing between them.   *4 marks*

Complete SAQs for Medical Finals By P. Stather et al, Published 2010 by Blackwell Publishing, ISBN: 978-1-4501-8928-6.

d In order to treat his ulcer you need to optimise his diabetic control. His is currently on one oral hypoglycaemic. Which would be best for him and why?   *2 marks*

e His BMs have been erratic, and you decide to start him on insulin. What HbA1c range are you aiming for?   *1 mark*

f Unfortunately his ulcer does not heal, and he develops ulcers on his toes, which have started to go black. Explain why this has happened.   *2 marks*

g These ulcers do not respond to medical treatment and require a below-knee amputation. Give two complications which may occur specifically related to this procedure.   *2 marks*

3 Eva is 74. She has been brought to A & E because she collapsed and hit her head when she stood up at church. Eva is known to have hypertension and arthritis and suffered an MI 3 years ago. Although Eva is conscious, she has no memory of what happened.

a Give four investigations, other than an ECG, that you would request, and state how the results may explain the collapse.   *8 marks*

b On ward round later in the day the consultant is concerned that you have not ruled out the possibility of Parkinson's disease as a common cause for collapse in the elderly. Give three signs of Parkinson's disease.   *3 marks*

c Why does Parkinson's disease occur?   *1 mark*

d Give two different classes of medical therapy you might employ in the treatment of patients with Parkinson's disease.   *2 marks*

4 Michael is 35. This is the second time he has presented to the surgical on take team complaining of severe pain and purulent discharge from the area around his anus. On examination around the anal area you find a small lump the size of a grape.

a Give two differential diagnoses.   *2 marks*

b As this is his second presentation with the same problem you are concerned that Michael may have an underlying predisposing medical problem such as Crohn's disease. Name one other medical condition that could be a predisposing factor in his presentation and state how you would test for it   *2 marks*

c Name three ways of differentiating between
   Crohn's disease and ulcerative colitis.   *3 marks*

d What three questions would you ask if you
   suspected inflammatory bowel disease?   *3 marks*

e What surgical treatment will be undertaken for
   Michael's current problem?   *1 mark*

f What medical treatment would you instigate for
   Crohn's disease?   *2 marks*

5 Joan, a 62-year-old lady, goes to see her GP for a review of her
blood pressure. She has been on medication for 6 months.

a How high must her BP be before you instigate
   medical therapy?   *1 mark*

b What two questions might you ask at this visit?   *2 marks*

c Name two complications of high blood pressure
   if left untreated.   *2 marks*

d If your hypertensive patient was a young lady,
   24 weeks pregnant, what two complications
   would you be concerned about?   *2 marks*

e On further questioning, this young lady
   explains that she is getting headaches and blurred
   vision. Her ankles are slightly oedematous.
   Her BP is 185/90. What is your immediate
   management?   *2 marks*

f Given the history, what two other investigations
   might you do?   *2 marks*

6 You are the surgical house officer on call and are referred Ewan,
a 22-year-old man who has a painful swollen left testicle.

a What is the most important diagnosis to rule out,
   and how does this condition occur?   *2 marks*

b State one further finding on examination
   which would lead you to believe this was the
   diagnosis.   *1 mark*

c Give three further causes of a swollen testicle.   *3 marks*

d You feel it is important to take a sexual
   history. Give three questions you would ask
   related to this.   *3 marks*

e You think this case may well be due to his
   promiscuity. You take swabs and a urine sample
   which shows a *Chlamydia* infection. Describe the
   optimum treatment for this.   *1 mark*

f Whilst examining him you suspect that he has a scrotal hernia. Explain how you can differentiate between a scrotal hernia and a swollen testicle. *1 mark*

g What is i) the anterior border of the inguinal canal and ii) the posterior border? *2 marks*

7 Kelly is an 8-year-old schoolgirl who suffers from asthma and is regularly admitted to hospital with exacerbations. In her last follow-up clinic you were very concerned about her asthma and were thinking about starting a long-term steroid to manage her condition.

a Name three other causes of dyspnoea in a child. *3 marks*

b Name two cells involved in the inflammatory response in asthma. *2 marks*

c Name three other types of drug used in the treatment of asthma and give an example of each. *3 marks*

d You want to measure her peak flow. How will you explain this to her? *2 marks*

e Name two drugs which can exacerbate asthma. *2 marks*

8 Martha is 56 and postmenopausal. She approaches you, her GP, reporting that she has felt a lump in her right breast. In her 20s she suffered from breast lumps which were cyclical in nature.

a What were the breast lumps in Martha's 20s likely to have been? *1 mark*

b What three further questions would you ask about the lump she presents with now? *3 marks*

c What three features will you look for on examination of the lump? *3 marks*

d What is peau d'orange? *1 mark*

e What is the commonest type of breast neoplasm? *1 mark*

f To which three organs does breast cancer typically metastasise? *3 marks*

g Give two mechanisms by which tumour metastasis may occur. *2 marks*

9 Margaret, a 68-year-old lady, comes to your outpatient clinic. Her GP has referred her to you as she presented 2 weeks ago after having suddenly found that she was blind in one eye. This lasted for a few hours. She did not have a headache. She has no other symptoms and no past medical history of note.

a What is the name given to Margaret's symptom?
What is the underlying cause? *2 marks*

b Name two important clinical signs you would
look for. *2 marks*

c Apart from blood tests, what three investigations
will you request? *3 marks*

d If, despite medical intervention, Margaret went
on to have a stroke, where is the most common
site of thromboembolism? *1 mark*

e Margaret was found to be in atrial fibrillation.
Name two important facets of her further
management. *2 marks*

f Where in the heart are clots likely to form in a
patient in AF? *1 mark*

10 Amy, a 10-year-old girl, presents with abdominal pain which
started centrally and has moved to the right iliac fossa. It has
been present for the past 2 days, and is associated with vomiting. She has no urinary or bowel symptoms.

a What is the most likely diagnosis? *1 mark*

b If she were 10 years older, what other important
diagnosis must you rule out? *1 mark*

c Given your suspected diagnosis, what would be
your initial management prior to seeking
senior advice? *3 marks*

d Your registrar reviews the patient and decides
to take her to theatre. Who may obtain consent
for this procedure? *1 mark*

e Suggest two people you may gain consent from
for this procedure. *2 marks*

f Before you get to theatre the pain spreads to the
rest of the abdomen. Your registrar becomes
more worried. Why? *1 mark*

g What surgical risks should this patient be
informed of prior to the procedure? Give four. *4 marks*

h Four days postoperatively her bowels have still
not opened. What is this called? *1 mark*

Practice Paper 2

ANSWERS

1 a Angina is caused by a decreased blood supply to heart *(1 mark)* due to poor coronary artery perfusion *(1 mark)*   `/2`

b During diastole *(1 mark)*   `/1`

c Decreases by more than 50% *(1 mark)* – the time taken for systole is 0.3 s, so with a pulse of 60 bpm there is 0.7 s for diastole. If the pulse rate doubles then there is only 0.2 s for diastole.   `/1`

d It is a vasodilator which acts predominantly on the veins thus reducing pre-load on the heart *(1 mark)*. It also causes dilatation of the coronary arteries *(1 mark)*   `/2`

e Long-acting nitrates, e.g. isosorbide mononitrate *(1 mark)*   `/1`

f Morphine *(1 mark)*   `/4`
GTN *(1 mark)*
Aspirin *(1 mark)*
Oxygen *(1 mark)*

g Lateral *(1 mark)*   `/1`

h Thrombolysis *(1 mark)*   `/2`
Angioplasty and stenting *(1 mark)*

2 a Weight/height × height = 120/1.7 × 1.7 = 41.5 *(1 mark)*   `/1`

b 20–25 *(1 mark)*   `/1`

c Neuropathic ulcer *(1 mark)* – sensory impairment causing deep painless ulcers. The foot will be warm with pulses present. There may be associated Charcot joints *(1 mark)*   `/4`
Ischaemic ulcer *(1 mark)* – will be painful and occur on toes and pressure points. The foot will often be cold with absent pulses, and the patient may suffer from claudication *(1 mark)*

d Metformin (biguanide) (*1 mark*) as it will help
with weight loss (*1 mark*) /2
e 6.5–7.5 (*1 mark*) /1
f The poor blood supply causes tissue necrosis /2
(*1 mark*), leading to gangrene (*1 mark*)
g (*maximum 2 marks*) /2
Phantom limb (*1 mark*)
Poor wound healing (*1 mark*)
Requirement for further amputation at a later
stage (*1 mark*)

3 a (*maximum 8 marks*) /8
FBC (*1 mark*) – low Hb could cause collapse
(*1 mark*)
U+E (*1 mark*) – deranged U+E may indicate
dehydration or electrolyte abnormalities as a
cause for collapse (*1 mark*)
CRP (*1 mark*) – high CRP indicates an infective
cause (*1 mark*)
Blood sugar (*1 mark*) – low blood glucose can
precipitate collapse (*1 mark*)
Urine dip and urinalysis (*1 mark*) – may show UTI
which can cause collapse in the elderly (*1 mark*)
Lying and standing blood pressure (*1 mark*) – postural
drop of 20 mmHg or more is abnormal (*1 mark*)
CXR (*1 mark*) – may demonstrate a pneumonia
which can lead to sepsis and collapse in the elderly
(*1 mark*)
CT head (*1 mark*) – presence of infarct or
haemorrhage, e.g. subdural haemorrhage
(*1 mark*)
b (*maximum 3 marks*) /3
Resting tremor of 4–7 Hz with pill-rolling
movements (*1 mark*)
Lead pipe rigidity (*1 mark*)
Cogwheeling (*1 mark*)
Bradykinesia (*1 mark*)
Typical stooped posture (*1 mark*)
Paucity of facial expression (*1 mark*)
Festinating gait (*1 mark*)
Dysarthria (*1 mark*)
Micrographia (*1 mark*)

c Parkinson's disease develops as a result of degeneration in the dopaminergic neurons of the substantia nigra, thus decreasing the amount of dopamine available *(1 mark)* `/1`

d *(maximum 2 marks)* `/2`
Dopamine antagonists – bromocriptine, pergolide *(1 mark)*
Levodopa *(1 mark)*
Monoamine oxidase B (MAOB) inhibitors – selegiline *(1 mark)*
Amantadine *(1 mark)*
Anticholinergics *(1 mark)*
Catechol-o-methyltransferase (COMT) inhibitors – entacapone *(1 mark)*

4 a *(maximum 2 marks)* `/2`
Perianal/ischiorectal abscess *(1 mark)*
Infected perianal varix *(1 mark)*
Fistula-in-ano *(1 mark)*
Anal cancer *(1 mark)*
Perianal Crohn's disease *(1 mark)*

b *(maximum 2 marks)* `/2`
Diabetes mellitus *(1 mark)* – random blood glucose level or OGTT *(1 mark)*
HIV *(1 mark)* – HIV antibody test, antigen test, or PCR *(1 mark)*

c Crohn's disease – characterised by skip lesions *(½ mark)*, can affect any area from mouth to anus *(½ mark)*, affects transmurally *(½ mark)* `/3`
Ulcerative colitis – characterised by full-thickness lesions progressing proximally from anus *(½ mark)*, affects colon only, although there may be some retrograde terminal ileitis *(½ mark)*, partial thickness *(½ mark)*

d *(maximum 3 marks)* `/3`
Has he passed any blood? *(1 mark)*
Has he passed any mucus? *(1 mark)*
How often is he having his bowels open each day? *(1 mark)*
Any weight loss? *(1 mark)*

e Incision and drainage *(1 mark)* `/1`

f *(maximum 2 marks)* ☐ /2
5-aminosalicylic acid (e.g. Pentasa) *(1 mark)*
High-dose short-course steroids in acute flares
    (1 mark)
Biological agents *(1 mark)*

5 a 160/95 on repeated readings (lower if she were ☐ /1
a diabetic) *(1 mark)*
 b Side-effects to current medications *(1 mark)* ☐ /2
Compliance with tablets *(1 mark)*
 c *(maximum 2 marks)* ☐ /2
Strokes *(1 mark)*
Aneurysms *(1 mark)*
MI *(1 mark)*
Angina *(1 mark)*
Renal failure *(1 mark)*
 d *(maximum 2 marks)* ☐ /2
Pre-eclampsia *(1 mark)*
Congenital anomalies in the foetus *(1 mark)*
Miscarriage *(1 mark)*
 e *(maximum 2 marks)* ☐ /2
Admit as emergency to Obstetrics *(1 mark)*
Complete rest *(1 mark)*
Start antihypertensive *(1 mark)*
 f *(maximum 2 marks)* ☐ /2
Dip urine to see if protein is present *(1 mark)*
Listen for baby's heart *(1 mark)*
Measure symphysis–fundal height to check baby is
    growing *(1 mark)*

6 a Testicular torsion *(1 mark)* ☐ /2
Twisting of the testicle leads to decreased blood
    supply to the testicle *(1 mark)*
 b *(maximum 1 mark)* ☐ /1
Extremely tender *(1 mark)*
Horizontal scrotum *(1 mark)*
Red scrotum *(1 mark)*
 c *(maximum 3 marks)* ☐ /3
Epididymitis *(1 mark)*
Inguinoscrotal hernia *(1 mark)*
Epididymal cyst *(1 mark)*
Hydrocoele *(1 mark)*

Testicular tumour *(1 mark)*

Varicocoele *(1 mark)*

Spermatocoele *(1 mark)*

d *(maximum 3 marks)* `/3`

Recent sexual partners *(1 mark)*

Any unprotected sexual intercourse *(1 mark)*

Trauma *(1 mark)*

Past infections *(1 mark)*

e Azithromycin 1 g stat *(1 mark)* `/1`

f You can get above a testicle, not a hernia `/1`
(1 mark)

g i) External oblique fascia *(1 mark)* `/1`

  ii) Inguinal ligament *(1 mark)* `/1`

7 a *(maximum 3 marks)* `/3`

Croup (*1 mark*)

Viral wheeze *(1 mark)*

Inhaled foreign body *(1 mark)*

Pneumonia *(1 mark)*

Pneumothorax *(1 mark)*

b *(maximum 2 marks)* `/2`

Mast cells *(1 mark)*

Eosinophils *(1 mark)*

Macrophages *(1 mark)*

Lymphocytes *(1 mark)*

c *(maximum 3 marks)* `/3`

B2 agonist, e.g. salbutamol (short-acting) or
salmeterol (long-acting) *(1 mark)*

Anticholinergic, e.g. ipratropium bromide
(1 mark)

Anti-inflammatories, e.g. sodium cromoglicate
(1 mark)

LTRA, e.g. montelukast *(1 mark)*

d *(maximum 2 marks)* `/2`

Ask her to breathe in as much as possible and then
to blow out quickly into the peak flow meter
(as if blowing out the candles on a birthday cake)
(1 mark). The device must be held horizontally
(1 mark). Lips must seal the mouthpiece tightly
(1 mark)

e NSAIDs *(1 mark)* `/2`

Beta-blocker *(1 mark)*

8 a Fibroadenomas *(1 mark)* `/1`

  b *(maximum 3 marks)* `/3`
How long has it been there? *(1 mark)*
Are there are any others? *(1 mark)*
Is it painful? *(1 mark)*
Does it change? *(1 mark)*
Is there any discharge from it? *(1 mark)*
Any skin changes? *(1 mark)*

  c *(maximum 3 marks)* `/3`
Any changes in the overlying skin *(1 mark)*
Size *(1 mark)*
Location *(1 mark)*
Consistency *(1 mark)*
Tethered to skin *(1 mark)*
Shape *(1 mark)*
Nipple discharge *(1 mark)*
Lymphadenopathy *(1 mark)*
Nipple abnormalities *(1 mark)*

  d Change in the skin overlying a carcinoma so that `/1`
it resembles the texture of orange skin *(1 mark)*

  e Adenocarcinoma *(1 mark)* `/1`

  f Lungs *(1 mark)* `/3`
Bones *(1 mark)*
Brain *(1 mark)*

  g *(maximum 2 marks)* `/2`
Direct invasion *(1 mark)*
Haematogenous spread *(1 mark)*
Lymphatic spread *(1 mark)*

9 a Amaurosis fugax *(1 mark)* `/2`
Caused by the passage of an embolus through
one of the retinal arteries *(1 mark)*

  b *(maximum 2 marks)* `/2`
Carotid artery bruit *(1 mark)*
AF *(1 mark)*
Evidence of valvular heart disease/endocarditis
(1 mark)

  c Echocardiogram *(1 mark)* `/3`
ECG *(1 mark)*
Carotid artery Doppler ultrasound
(1 mark)

  d Middle cerebral artery *(1 mark)* `/1`

e *(maximum 2 marks)* `/2`
Anticoagulation – usually with warfarin *(1 mark)*
Digoxin if pulse rate >100 *(1 mark)*
Rate control – beta-blockers *(1 mark)*
Cardioversion *(1 mark)*
Radiofrequency ablation of accessory pathways
 (1 mark)
f The left atrial appendage *(1 mark)* `/1`

10 a Appendicitis *(1 mark)* `/1`
 b Ectopic pregnancy *(1 mark)* `/1`
 c *(maximum 3 marks)* `/3`
 NBM *(1 mark)*
 Cannula and IV fluids *(1 mark)*
 Bloods (FBC, U+E, CRP, clotting, group and save)
  (1 mark)
 Urine dip and culture *(1 mark)*
 d *(maximum 1 mark)* `/1`
 Any doctor capable of performing the procedure
 (1 mark) or a nominated person who is suitably
 trained/qualified and has sufficient knowledge of
 the proposed procedure and the risks involved
 (see GMC guidance) *(1 mark)*
 e *(maximum 2 marks)* `/2`
 The child (if Fraser competent) *(1 mark)*
 The mother *(1 mark)*
 The father if the parents were married at the time
  of birth *(1 mark)*
 f The appendix is likely to have perforated *(1 mark)* `/1`
 g *(maximum 4 marks)* `/4`
 Bleeding *(1 mark)*
 Infection *(1 mark)*
 Urinary retention *(1 mark)*
 Ileus *(1 mark)*
 Adhesions *(1 mark)*
 Postoperative pain *(1 mark)*
 Perforation of bowel *(1 mark)*
 Anaesthetic risks *(1 mark)*
 h Ileus *(1 mark)* `/1`

Abbreviations

5-ASA	5-aminosalicylic acid
AAFB	Acid and alcohol-fast bacilli
A & E	Accident and Emergency Department
ABC	Airway, breathing, circulation
ABG	Arterial blood gas
ABPI	Ankle brachial pressure index
ACEI	Angiotensin converting enzyme inhibitor
ACL	Anterior cruciate ligament
ACTH	Adrenocorticotrophic hormone
ADL	Activities of daily living
AF	Atrial fibrillation
AIDS	Acquired immunodeficiency disorder
ALL	Acute lymphocytic leukaemia
ALT	Alanine aminotransferase
AML	Acute myeloid leukaemia
ANA	Antinuclear antibody
ANCA	Antinuclear cytoplasmic antibody
Anti-CCP	Anti-cyclic citrullinated peptide
AP	Anteroposterior
ARDS	Adult respiratory distress syndrome
ARF	Acute renal failure
ARMD	Age related macular degeneration
ASAP	As soon as possible
AST	Aspartate transaminase
AXR	Abdominal x-ray
BCC	Basal cell carcinoma
BD	Twice per day
BMI	Body mass index
BMs	Boehringer Mannheim (blood sugar monitoring strips)
BP	Blood pressure
BMP	Beats per minute
BPH	Benign prostatic hypertrophy

BTS	British Thoracic Society
CABG	Coronary artery bypass graft
CBD	Common bile duct
CBT	Cognitive behavioural therapy
CCU	Coronary Care Unit
CJD	Creutzfeldt–Jakob disease
CLL	Chronic lymphocytic leukaemia
CML	Chronic myeloid leukaemia
CMV	Cytomegalovirus
CNS	Central nervous system
COCP	Combined oral contraceptive pill
COMT	Catechol-o-methyl transferase
CPR	Cardiopulmonary resuscitation
Cr	Creatinine
CREST	calcinosis, Raynaud's disease, oesophagitis, sclerodactyly, telangiectasia
CRF	Chronic renal failure
CRP	C-reactive protease
CSF	Cerebrospinal fluid
CT	Computed tomography scan
CTG	Cardiotocograph
CTPA	Computerised tomographic pulmonary angiogram
CVA	Cerebrovascular accident
CXR	Chest x-ray
DIC	Disseminated intravascular coagulation
DMARDs	Disease-modifying anti-rheumatic drugs
DVT	Deep vein thrombosis
EBV	Epstein Barr virus
ECG	Electrocardiogram
ECHO	Echocardiogram
EEG	Electroencephalogram
eGFR	Estimated glomerular filtration rate
EMG	Electromyography
ENT	Ear, nose and throat
EPS	Extrapyramidal symptom
ERCP	Endoscopic retrograde cholangeopancreatography
ESR	Erythrocyte sedimentation rate
FAP	Familial adenomatous polyposis
FBC	Full blood count
FNA	Fine needle aspirate
FSH	Follicle-stimulating hormone

GCS	Glasgow coma score
GGT	Gamma-glutamyl transpeptidase
GI	Gastrointestinal
GIFT	Gamete intrafallopian transfer
GORD	Gastro-oesophageal reflux disease
GP	General practitioner
GTN	Glyceryl trinitrate
GU	Genitourinary
H2RA	H2 receptor antagonist
HAART	Highly active antiretroviral therapy
Hb	Haemoglobin
HbA1c	Glycosylated haemoglobin
bHCG	Beta human chorionic gonadotropin
HELLP	Haemolytic anaemia, elevated liver enzymes and low platelet count
HiB	Haemophilus influenza B
HIV	Human immunodeficiency virus
HLA	Human leukocytes antigen
HNPCC	Hereditary non-polyposis colorectal cancer
HOCM	Hypertrophic obstructive cardiomyopathy
HPV	Human papilloma virus
HRCT	High resolution computed tomography
HRT	Hormone replacement therapy
HSV	Herpes simplex virus
IBS	Irritable bowel syndrome
ICU	Intensive Care Unit
IgA	Immunoglobulin type A
IgG	Immunoglobulin type G
IgM	Immunoglobulin type M
IM	Intramuscular
INR	International standardised ratio
IUCD	Intrauterine contraceptive device
IUGR	Intrauterine growth retardation
IV	Intravenous
IVF	In vitro fertilisation
IVP	Intravenous pyelogram
ISMN	Isosorbide mononitrate
K	Potassium
LDH	Lactate dehydrogenase
L-dopa	Levodopa
LFT	Liver function tests
LH	Luteinising hormone

LHRH	Luteinising hormone releasing hormone
LLQ	Left lower quadrant
LMP	Last menstrual period
LMWH	Low molecular-weight heparin
LUQ	Left upper quadrant
LUTs	Lower urinary tract symptoms
MALT	Mucosa-associated lymphoid tissue
MAOI	Monoamine oxidase inhibitor
MC+S	Microscopy, culture and sensitivities
MCV	Mean corpuscular volume
MGUS	Monoclonal gammaopathy of unknown specificity
MI	Myocardial infarction
MMR	Measles, mumps and rubella
MMSE	Mini mental state examination
MRI	Magnetic resonance imaging
MS	Multiple sclerosis
MSU	Midstream urine
Na	Sodium
NBM	Nil by mouth
NG	Nasogastric
NHL	Non-Hodgkin's lymphoma
NICE	National Institute for Clinical Excellence
NIV	Non-invasive ventilation
NMDA	N-methyl-D-aspartic acid
NOF	Neck of femur
NSAIDs	Non-steroidal anti-inflammatory drugs
NSTEMI	Non-ST elevation myocardial infarction
NYHA	New York Heart Association
OCD	Obsessive compulsive disorder
OCP	Oral contraceptive pill
OD	Once per day
O/E	On examination
OGD	Oesophagogastroduodenoscopy
OGGT	Oral glucose tolerance test
OPD	Outpatients department
OT	Occupational therapy
PCKD	Polycystic kidney disease
PCOS	Polycystic ovarian syndrome
PE	Pulmonary embolism
PEFR	Peak expiratory flow rate
PEG	Percutaneous enterogastrotomy

PET scan	Positron emission tomography
PID	Pelvic inflammatory disease
Plts	Platelets
PMH	Past medical history
PPI	Proton pump inhibitor
PR	Per rectum
PRN	As required
PROM	Premature rupture of membranes
PUJ	Pelviureteric junction
PUVA	Photosensitive ultraviolet light
PV	Per vagina
PVD	Peripheral vascular disease
QDS	Four times per day
RA	Rheumatoid arthritis
Rh	Rhesus
RICE	Rest, ice, compress, elevate
RIF	Right iliac fossa
RLQ	Right lower quadrant
RR	Respiratory rate
RSV	Respiratory syncytial virus
RUQ	Right upper quadrant
SAH	Subarachnoid haemorrhage
SALT	Speech and language therapy
SAU	Surgical Admissions Unit
S/C	Subcutaneous
S/L	Sublingual
SLE	Systemic lupus erythematosus
SOB	Short of breath
SSRI	Selective serotonin reuptake inhibitor
SNRI	Serotonin noradrenaline reuptake inhibitor
STEMI	ST elevation myocardial infarction
STI	Sexually transmitted infection
SUFE	Slipped upper femoral epiphysis
TAH+BSO	Total abdominal hysterectomy and bilateral salpingo-oopherectomy
TB	Tuberculosis
TDS	Three times per day
TFT	Thyroid function test
TIA	Transient ischaemic attack
TENS	Transcutaneous electrical nerve stimulation
TNM	Tumour, nodes, metastases
TOP	Termination of pregnancy

TORCH	Toxoplasmosis, other agents, rubella, cytomegalovirus and herpes simplex
TURP	Transurethral resection of prostate
TSH	Thyroid stimulating hormone
U+E	Urea and electrolytes
UC	Ulcerative colitis
Ur	Urea
USS	Ultrasound scan
UTI	Urinary tract infection
VE	Vaginal examination
vWF	Von Willebrand's factor
VZV	Varicella zoster virus
WCC	White cell count
ZIFT	Zygote intrafallopian transfer

Reference Ranges

Haemoglobin (men)	13–18 g/dL
(women)	11.5–16 g/dL
Mean cell volume	76–96 fL
Platelets	150–400 × 10^9/L
White cells (total)	4–11 × 10^9/L
Neutrophils	1.8–7.5 × 10^9/L
Sodium	135–145 mmol/L
Potassium	3.5–5.0 mmol/L
Urea	2.5–6.7 mmol/L
Creatinine	70–150 µmol/L
Calcium	2.12–2.65 mmol/L
Bilirubin	3–17 µmol/L
Alanine aminotransferase (ALT)	3–35 IU/L
Aspartate transaminase (AST)	3–35 IU/L
Alkaline phosphatase	30–35 IU/L
Albumin	35–50 g/L
Amylase	0–180 Somogyi U/dL
CRP	<5 mg/L
Fasting glucose	3.5–5.5 mmol/L
Total thyroxine (T4)	70–140 mol/L
Thyroid stimulating hormone	0.5–5 mU/L
pH	7.35–7.45
PaO_2	>10.6
$PaCO_2$	4.7–6.0
Base excess	± 2 mmol/L